DENIAL

Also by Dan Olmsted and Mark Blaxill

The Age of Autism: Mercury, Medicine, and a Man-made Epidemic

Vaccines 2.0: The Careful Parent's Guide to Making Safe Vaccination Choices For Your Family

By Mark Blaxill

The Invisible Edge: Taking Your Strategy to the Next Level Using Intellectual Property

DENIAL

How Refusing to Face the Facts
about Our Autism Epidemic Hurts
Children, Families, and Our Future

BY DAN OLMSTED AND MARK BLAXILL

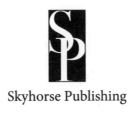

Skyhorse Publishing

DEDICATION

To Bernard Rimland
Who sought the truth and helped sick kids

Skyhorse Publishing books may be purchased in bulk at special discounts for sales promotion, corporate gifts, fund-raising, or educational purposes. Special editions can also be created to specifications. For details, contact the Special Sales Department, Skyhorse Publishing, 307 West 36th Street, 11th Floor, New York, NY 10018 or info@ skyhorsepublishing.com.

Skyhorse® and Skyhorse Publishing® are registered trademarks of Skyhorse Publishing, Inc.®, a Delaware corporation.

Visit our website at www.skyhorsepublishing.com.

10 9 8 7 6 5 4 3 2 1

Library of Congress Cataloging-in-Publication Data is available on file.

Cover design by Rain Saukas

Print ISBN: 978–1–5107–1694–0
Ebook ISBN: 978–1–5107–1695–7

Printed in the United States of America

Contents

"Over half of all American children* now suffer from chronic illnesses in numbers unheard of just a few short years ago. The fact that this is not the biggest story in America is proof of the willful ignorance of government and main stream media."

—Rob Schneider, actor

---

*   http://www.sciencedirect.com/science/article/pii/S1876285910002500

Dramatis Personae

Autism Discoverers

1. Leo Kanner, child psychiatrist at Johns Hopkins Hospital in Baltimore and author of the 1943 paper, "Autistic Disturbances of Affective Contact," that first described eleven children with what came to be known as early infantile autism.
2. Hans Asperger, pediatrician in Vienna and author of the 1944 paper, "Autistic Pathology in Childhood." It contained four case histories of what came to be known as Asperger's syndrome.

Psychiatry Pioneers

1. Emil Kraepelin, German founder of modern psychiatry who in the late nineteenth century systematized mental illness under "affective" and "psychotic" categories, the latter including *dementia praecox*, a psychotic illness of adolescence and early adulthood.
2. Eugen Bleuler, German psychiatrist who in the early twentieth century renamed *dementia praecox* "schizophrenia" and coined the term "autismus" for the isolated and self-involved trait evident in schizophrenia. The word was later adopted by Kanner and Asperger to describe the extreme isolation of the new disorders they were describing.

3. Adolf Meyer, Kanner's mentor at Johns Hopkins, who along with Dr. Esther Richards saw a child, Jane, that Kanner believed was autistic—if so, a very early case description.
4. Irwin Lazar, founder and director of the Viennese children's health clinic where Asperger, Homberger, Frankl, and Weiss worked. Student of Bleuler.

Observers of Childhood Psychoses

1. D. Arn van Krevelen, Dutch psychiatrist and early observer of autism and Asperger's, which, he argued, were distinct syndromes.
2. Theodor Heller, discoverer of what is now called Childhood Disintegrative Disorder in Vienna in 1907. Often called Heller's disease, Heller-Weygandt syndrome, or *dementia infantilis*.
3. Wilhelm Weygandt, who saw one of Heller's patients, a four-year-old boy, and wrote about it in a Viennese medical journal in 1907.
4. Sante De Sanctis, Italian doctor who described a disorder similar to Heller-Weygandt's he called *dementia praecocisemia*.
5. Julius Zappert, leading Viennese child psychiatrist who confirmed Heller's observations of rare cases of childhood disintegrative disorders throughout Europe.
6. Grunya Sukhareva, Russian psychiatrist who observed "schizoid" (eccentric) children in Moscow in the 1920s in what appears to be the earliest description of "Little Professor" or Asperger-type children.
7. Georg Frankl, chief diagnostician in the Vienna clinic who came to the United States and helped examine Case 1, Donald T., in Leo Kanner's landmark paper. Silberman speculates Frankl told Kanner about Asperger's autism discoveries and Kanner stole them.
8. Anni Weiss, doctor in Vienna clinic who, in 1936, described a child, Gottfried, who may have been first "Little Professor" case reported in Europe. Married Frankl in the United States after both fled the Nazis.
9. Franz Hamburger, head of the University Hospital of Vienna; Asperger's boss with Nazi sympathies who may nevertheless have shielded him from the Nazis.

10. August Homburger, Viennese psychiatrist who wrote a text on childhood psychiatric conditions but mentioned only Weygandt and Heller, not a syndrome similar to autism.

11. Howard Potter, American psychiatrist who wrote a definitive article on childhood schizophrenics in 1933 that contained no mention of a condition comparable to early infantile autism.

12. E. E. Grebelskaya-Albatz, Russian psychiatrist who reported in mid-1930s on cases of Heller's and early-onset schizophrenia but no syndrome similar to autism.

13. Jakob Lutz, wrote case description of "Otto," born in 1923. His symptoms began early enough to be consistent with autism, but other features did not match. Lutz called it "an insidiously progressive early form of childhood psychosis."

14. Herbert Jancke, German doctor who in 1929 presented a case history called "Girl" of a child who regressed before age two.

15. N. Moritz Tramer, author of multipart "Diary About a Mentally Ill Child," based on his mother's diaries, perhaps the most complete account of regression in infancy. The child, known as "P," might have had any number of conditions, possibly including mercury poisoning from "gray powder" used to treat diarrhea.

16. Lightner Witmer, Philadelphia psychiatrist who wrote in 1920 about a child, Don, with symptoms that autism pioneer Bernard Rimland considered autistic; but post-pertussis encephalitis in infancy is alternate explanation.

17. Mildred Creak, British doctor who wrote about "Psychoses in Children" in 1937; nothing resembling autism is cited.

18. R. A. Q. Lay, London doctor whose review paper on "Psychoses in Children" in 1938 is the most exhaustive account of childhood mental illnesses up to that date (the same year the first autistic child, Donald T., was seen at Kanner's Baltimore clinic). Serves as bulwark against the idea that syndromes similar to autism had always been around.

19. Esther Richards, psychiatrist who worked with Kanner and spotted one of his eleven cases, Virginia S., in a home for the "feeble-minded." Remarked that she stood out as "completely different" from others in the home.

20. Louise Despert, New York City Freudian child psychiatrist who took issue with Kanner that his cases represented a new syndrome but eventually concluded they did.

21. Lauretta Bender, whose 1947 paper "Childhood Schizophrenia" was the first after Kanner's 1943 paper to capture children with regression during infancy—autism.

22. J. Franklin Robinson, coauthor in 1954 of "Children With Restricted Interests," first paper in America to describe children with clear Asperger's syndrome.

23. Louis J. Vitale, coauthor of above paper with J. Franklin Robinson. He and Robinson were doctors at a clinic in Wilkes-Barre, Pennsylvania.

Earlier Observers of Mental Disorders, Including Children

1. Samuel Gridley Howe, conducted thorough study of intellectually disabled people in Massachusetts in 1848, found a handful that Donvan and Zucker believe show autism was present that far back.

2. John Haydon Langdon Down, discoverer of Down syndrome whose further studies turned up children some believe were autistic but may have been genetically susceptible to environmental damage.

3. William Wotherspoon Ireland, whose book *On Idiocy and Imbecility* in 1898 looked at insane children but found none that would fit the definition of autism.

4. Alfred Frank Tredgold, whose book *Mental Deficiency* also looked at insanity in children but found nothing like autism.

5. John Haslam, chief apothecary of the Bethlem Asylum, whose 1809 Monograph, *Observations on Madness and Melancholy,* reported on two children who were plausibly autistic, both of whom surfaced following vaccination reactions.

6. Henry Maudsley, whose 1807 book *The Pathology and Physiology of the Mind* covered insanity in early life but turned up nothing like autism.

7. Jean-Etienne Esquirol, pioneer French doctor in diagnosis and treatment of insanity in France who, in an 1845 book, observed that mental illness was absent in infancy, a direct refutation of the claim autism was always present since it must manifest in infancy.
8. Richard Napier, "family doctor" in London around 1600, among whose clientele mentally ill children were "strikingly rare."
9. William Howship Dickinson, at Great Ormond Street Hospital for Children, who kept careful records of children's medical problems; later examination found three whose symptoms match autism.

Prologue: Waiting

here were they?
        From his child psychiatry practice in Holland, D. Arn van Krevelen watched. And waited. He had been on the lookout now for almost a decade.

The year was 1952. During his career, van Krevelen had seen just about every variety of mental disorder. He diagnosed teenagers developing the first signs of schizophrenia; he saw brain damage from injury and illness; he witnessed the sudden psychic disintegration of children known as *dementia infantilis*. Now he was watching for something different—"markedly and uniquely different from anything reported so far," as the first child psychiatrist to observe it wrote in 1943.

These children shared "fascinating peculiarities"—unusual use of language, or none at all; rituals centered on objects and obsessions; lack of emotional connection with parents or any other human beings. They should be easy to spot: they were, after all, unique. Yet, van Krevelen was starting to doubt their existence.

Where were they? Where were the children with autism?[1]

Introduction: "What Hump?"

E ven as the autism toll passes a million children[2] and the cost soars to a trillion dollars,[3] a pernicious idea is taking hold: there simply is no autism epidemic.

The implications are enormous. Is autism ancient, a genetic variation that begs only for overdue acceptance and acknowledgment? Or is it recent and growing, the frightening product of something toxic to which our children are succumbing?

We believe autism *is* new and the rate really has risen dramatically. "Autism is a public health crisis of historic proportions," one of us testified to a Congressional Committee in December 2012.[4] Therefore, we as a nation face an obligation to take urgent action against an epidemic of disability that too many "experts" won't acknowledge, don't take seriously, or simply deny. They are flat earthers for the new millennium. We call them Epidemic Deniers. They do nothing but confuse the facts about a clear-cut, man-made catastrophe and, unconscionably, delay the day of reckoning and response.

We have learned these truths from our own experience and seen them confirmed day in and day out for many years. One of us is the parent of a daughter with an autism diagnosis who will never live independently. The other has reported on autism for a decade and watched the rate soar even in that short period. Together, we wrote *The Age of Autism* in 2010, delving deeper into its natural history than ever before, and identifying eight of the first eleven cases in the medical literature, including Case 1, Donald T., whom we visited at his child-hood home in Mississippi where he still resides. Those first cases were reported in 1943,[5] a mere tick on history's timepiece.

Yet today a million and more Americans, almost all of them under thirty, have been formally diagnosed with autism. Yes, it is a spectrum disorder, but variation should not confuse the issue. Most with an autism diagnosis will never be employed, pay taxes, fall in love, get married, have children, or be responsible for their health and welfare. Both the increase and the burden it imposes are widely recognized by thousands of parents and frontline professionals such as nurses and teachers. Yet some of the most prominent and powerful people in medicine, the media, and government deny it.

Rejecting this reality is itself a kind of disorder—Epidemic Denial. It is a little like bug-eyed Marty Feldman as a hunchback in *Young Frankenstein,* responding to Gene Wilder's Count Frankenstein with the indignant, "What hump?" It's the Big Lie about autism. But instead of fading as more and more evidence reveals the scope and scale of autism's effect on American children, Epidemic Denial is gaining trac-tion, especially from two books that slickly package false logic, weak data, and syrupy nostrums to argue against the very existence of an epidemic.

" . . . Autistic people have always been part of the human commu-nity, though they have often been relegated to the margins of society," writes Steve Silberman in *NeuroTribes: The Legacy of Autism and the Future of Neurodiversity.*[6]

No, they have not. While autistic traits may always have been part of the human profile, their severity and ubiquity have not, and the *dis-ability* of those with autism is what keeps the vast majority at the mar-gins of society.

John Donvan and Caren Zucker, the authors of *In a Different Key: The History of Autism,* are dubious about an epidemic but dodge the issue in a way that makes it seem trivial rather than existential. "We don't really know if there is not an epidemic, but we also think that it shouldn't matter when we decide whether or not to respond to the needs of people in the autism community," says Donvan, an ABC News reporter.[7] "It shouldn't matter whether there's an epidemic or not."

Yes, it should. And yes, there is.

Donvan and Zucker are of course right about responding to the needs of those with autism. But they're dead wrong that the epidemic question doesn't really matter. How, for one thing, do you plan for the needs of twenty-one-year-olds a decade hence if you don't concede their numbers will have greatly increased?

Autism Epidemic Denial belongs in the fiction category. Yet both books have been widely acclaimed. A "magnificent opus," the *Washington Post* said of *In a Different Key*.[8] "A tour de force of archival, journalistic and scientific research, both scholarly and widely accessible," said chief judge Anne Applebaum of *NeuroTribes*, the first popular science book to win Britain's prestigious Samuel Johnson Prize (and $35,000).[9] Mainstream reviewers have proven themselves too indoctrinated, too uninterested, or too incurious to question the dubious premise of these books, which are presented in dulcet tones that echo today's cultural memes of inclusivity and self-advocacy. Not that anything is wrong with that—but it's only half the story, the half that screenwriters and TV news segments love to showcase. In the real world, the autism rate is up one hundredfold in the three decades (see

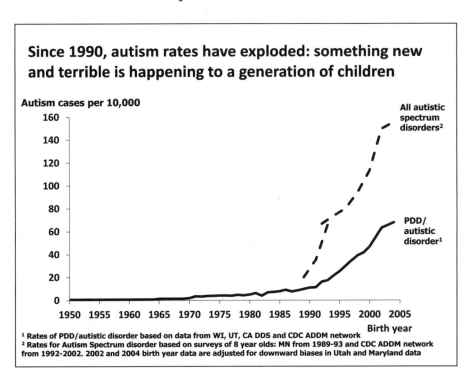

Since 1990, autism rates have exploded: something new and terrible is happening to a generation of children

Autism cases per 10,000

All autistic spectrum disorders[2]

PDD/autistic disorder[1]

Birth year

[1] Rates of PDD/autistic disorder based on data from WI, UT, CA DDS and CDC ADDM network
[2] Rates for Autism Spectrum disorder based on surveys of 8 year olds: MN from 1989-93 and CDC ADDM network from 1992-2002. 2002 and 2004 birth year data are adjusted for downward biases in Utah and Maryland data

chart) with a clear inflection point around 1990, pointing to environmental exposures, not better detection or broader diagnosis.

Even the CDC, charged with determining the autism rate, is blandly agnostic. "Is there an ASD [autism spectrum disorder] epidemic?" the agency asks on its autism page. "A: More people than ever before are being diagnosed with an ASD. It is unclear exactly how much of this increase is due to a broader definition of ASD and better efforts in diagnosis. However, a true increase in the number of people with an ASD cannot be ruled out. We believe the increase in the diagnosis of ASD is likely due to a combination of these factors."[10]

That's mush.

Hence, this book. The case against Epidemic Denial is convincing, and we intend to make it forcefully and fully. Upon close examination, Epidemic Denial is not merely improbable or implausible but *impossible*. The Deniers' argument falls into a number of logic traps and evidence gaps so deep it can't get up. Epidemic Deniers simply have not put their ideas to the tests they must survive in order to be taken seriously. We'll use key evidence from medical history to demonstrate what we mean.

We will show that before 1930, the rate of autism was effectively zero. The rise was slow at first—van Krevelen was looking for the first autism case as late as 1952—but by the late 1980s, it began to accelerate sharply and has since become a feature of life in every community. Last year, educators in Minneapolis announced plans for a high school exclusively for students with an autism diagnosis;[11] a toy store for autistic children opened recently in Chicago.[12] Yet we are to believe this level of special education, this need for accommodation, was present all along and just now provided.

We call bullshit on that.

◆ ◆ ◆

Epidemic denial doesn't add up. Take the US population of 124 million in 1931—the year the eldest child in that first report on autism was born. Divide that number by the current autism prevalence of one in sixty-eight children. There should have been 1.8 million Americans with autism in 1931.

There weren't. We have scoured the medical literature for cases before then, and there are essentially none to be found. This may seem counterintuitive—surely such children have always been around, misdiagnosed by a less sophisticated medical establishment or simply missed because they were hidden away in an attic or mental institution—but it's the simple truth.

Back up a bit more: how many people have ever lived on Earth? About 100 billion by 1931. Again, simple math yields about one-and-a-half billion autistic individuals who have lived before 1930.

Now we begin to glimpse the emptiness behind the Epidemic Denier's claims. There may have been scattered individuals with enough traits to qualify for an autism diagnosis, but 1.5 billion would have been far more visible. Someone would have said something. Given the distinctive profile of autistic children, it's impossible that no doctor or social observer commented on their markedly different behavior.

Now zoom in again and consider the population of Forest, Mississippi, where Case 1, Donald Triplett, was born in 1933. As Jonathan Rose, a history professor at Drew University, points out, at today's rate of one in sixty-eight children, there should have been sixty autistic people back then in that small town of three thousand. Donald would have been one of many with similar profiles. There would have been adults, special classes, and dozens of autistic people roaming the streets alongside Donald. Instead, he was an oddity never seen before.

Clearly, he was alone.

So why claim otherwise in the face of both common sense and clear data? Some just *assume* a condition as well entrenched as autism must always have been around, with the well-known consequences of *ass*uming anything. Others suspect the increase is only too real but find no reason to upset the status quo, the circular round of benefits, grants, breathless gene "breakthroughs" of no real significance—and back to benefits.

And too many *do* know but let the epidemic roll on in the service of something sinister—saving their reputations, avoiding liability, making money, and in some cases ducking potential criminal liability. They put their careers ahead of our kids. We are not conspiracy theorists; we don't need to be when so much has been placed in the public record in the past few years.

The question is *cui bono*—who benefits?

◆ ◆ ◆

Autism is simply not a feel-good story; it is not about research advances, better understanding, or misunderstood geniuses. The toll of disability from autism rapidly erodes our standing in the world and adds billions to educational services that are already strained. At one prominent US high school with more than three thousand students whose data the authors reviewed confidentially, one in forty-nine has an autism diagnosis—and even then the most severe cases are receiving educational services off-campus and not counted in that total.

◆ ◆ ◆

Like Neapolitan ice cream, Epidemic Denial comes in three flavors. There's something to suit the tastes of different audiences—inclusion, diversity, evidence of medical prowess, hidden aptitudes, a wonderful next step in evolution we can barely imagine.

Flavor One wants us to believe that "science," like some kind of omniscient god, rejects claims of an epidemic. Doctors and the medical field in general love this flavor because it reflects admirably on their powers of observation compared to earlier generations. It fits with the march of medical progress conquering all before it. Michael Crichton, the great popular fiction writer who was also a Harvard-trained MD, took this idea apart as well as anyone we know.

"Let's be clear: the work of science has nothing whatever to do with consensus," he wrote. "Consensus is the business of politics. Science, on the contrary, requires only one investigator who happens to be right, which means that he or she has results that are verifiable by reference to the real world."

The overall theme of the Deniers is that the so-called autism epidemic is an artifact of better diagnosis. "It's not an actual epidemic," as vaccine researcher and patent holder and de facto Denier-in-Chief Paul Offit put it. "In the mid-1990s, the definition of autism was broadened to what is now called autism spectrum disorder. People say if you took the current criteria and went back 50 years, you'd see about as many children with autism then."[13] No, people don't say that. They say they waited years for the first sighting, like van Krevelen in Holland. Medical students into the 1970s and '80s here and abroad gathered round to see a single autistic patient. They were told it might be the only such case in their careers.

The better-diagnosis claim incorporates three elements. One is diagnostic *substitution*—children previously diagnosed as mentally retarded, for example, now getting a primary diagnosis of autism. The second is diagnostic *expansion*, in which, say, the inclusion of Asperger's syndrome on the autism spectrum in 1994 attracted a new cohort of less-severe cases that were previously considered eccentric, not diagnosable. The third is diagnostic *oversight*, in which hordes of people who should have had an autism diagnosis were simply overlooked.

Offit's claim is pure diagnostic expansion. Silberman's argument in *NeuroTribes* is substitution: "For most of the twentieth century, they [autistic people] were hidden behind a welter of competing labels— Sukhareva's 'schizoid personality disorder,' Despert and Bender's 'childhood schizophrenia,' Robinson and Vitale's 'children with circumscribed interests,' [Temple] Grandin's initial diagnosis of 'minimal brain damage,' and many other labels not mentioned in this book, such as 'multiplex personality disorder,' which have fallen out of use."[14] Zucker and Donvan are big on diagnostic oversight, pointing to holy fools, village savants, and feral children as examples as people who were never counted as part of the autism family.

All this sounds reasonable, but it's demonstrably wrong, and that's what matters. Better diagnosing can't account for a fraction of the well-documented twentyfold increase we've seen over just the past two decades. Our colleague J. B. Handley calls Epidemic Denial the "original sin" of autism. "In Offit's world, there is absolutely *no problem here.* Things are as they always were, we just understand it better. Of course, we all know, if there's no epidemic, there is no environmental trigger, because why have a trigger if something hasn't actually grown? Said differently: Denying the autism epidemic is to deny the suffering of millions of children and their families and also to deny the exploration into the true cause so the epidemic might end."[15]

To persist in this folly requires not just abdicating common sense— *Who are you going to believe, Epidemic Deniers or your own lying eyes?*—but ignoring more and more evidence. For instance: In 2009, researchers at the University of California at Davis MIND Institute found "the seven- to eightfold increase in the number of children born in California with autism since 1990 cannot be explained by either changes in how the condition is diagnosed or counted—and the trend shows no sign of abating."[16] The findings, which appeared in the journal *Epidemiology,* "also suggest that research should shift from genetics to the host of chemicals and infectious microbes in the environment that are likely at the root of changes in the neurodevelopment of California's children."

◆ ◆ ◆

Flavor Two of Epidemic Denial wants us not only to believe that autism has always been with us, but also that it is mild and useful to society. Silberman: "Asperger's lost tribe finally emerged from the shadows" to launch all sorts of modern inventions.

A lost tribe of high-functioning, technically gifted individuals with autism whose contribution to the modern world is at long last being recognized? Hardly. Here it's important to distinguish between autistic traits, such as repetitive rocking or delayed speech, and the diagnosis of Autistic Disorder. Such traits are simply *not* the same as an autism diagnosis, which requires evidence of significant problems with communication, restricted interests, and social isolation, all by a child's third birthday. So you can be a nerd or a geek, transfixed by a special topic or possessing savant skills, yet be nowhere near meeting the criteria for the autism spectrum.

Those traits may be exemplified or taken to their extreme by autistic people, but a "dusting" of one of them does not make a person eligible for a disability diagnosis; there is such a thing as human variation that is not pathological. Having traits that are similar to the autism checklist is not autism.

For Silberman, Hans Asperger in Vienna is the hero. He discovered and nurtured the precocious "Little Professors" whose syndrome would eventually bear his name, while in Baltimore the cold and ambitious Leo Kanner focused solely on severe cases and stole credit that was rightly Asperger's. This kind of biased biography serves

Silberman's purposes, but it's a speculative mishmash. Neither Kanner nor Asperger were perfect, but they did the world a service by reporting what they saw with detail that has never been surpassed.

NeuroTribes also taps into the phenomenon of people who self-identify as autistic as adults. This trend of "neurodiversity" deserves skepticism, not because it empowers people to make the most of their circumstances—that's great—but because it is so often used to clobber those of us who believe that autism is an environmental injury, most often disabling, that calls for action. Many such self-diagnosed advocates are suspect. Adults who went to school, got married, started families and successful careers—and then belatedly decided they are autistic—don't seem terribly disabled. One self-described self-advocate, Michael John Carley, accomplished all that and more, and those who have seen him in public regard him as an intelligent and articulate person who can play political games with the best of them. He began his presentation to a congressional committee in 2012 by saying that because he was autistic he needed more time than other speakers to express himself, a clever move that almost screams *"not* autistic!"[17]

Is that the same as a child who can't go to school, can't speak, let alone get married or participate in the complex identity politics of American society? It is not, even if it comes from a loving place of identifying with an autistic child. There's no reason to believe Carley has zero autistic traits. But there's also no reason to believe he would have qualified for a disability diagnosis based on behaviors evident in infancy, as an ASD requires.

By definition, autistic people, or at least the most disabled that constitute the core of the autism crisis, can't advocate for themselves. For the Michael John Carleys of the autism self-advocacy world to step in and take a voice away from parents of such profoundly disabled children is unjustified. But it's just the kind of climate Silberman, Donvan, Zucker, Offit, and the rest of the Epidemic Denial crowd encourage and enable.

◆ ◆ ◆

Flavor Three is exemplified by Donvan and Zucker's *In a Different Key;* they can't be bothered to either confirm or deny an autism epidemic even as they dismiss or neglect most of the evidence that supports it.

These authors—who have autism in their family—are more realistic about its severity in the vast majority of cases. But their argument is the least serious, an emotional soufflé of good feelings and "person of the week" happy talk that collapses like soufflés so often do. (The book evolved from scripts of ABC News autism segments they produced, and it reads that way. The glowing *Washington Post* review begins: "I was on Page 86 . . . when I began casting the movie.")[18] Like savvy Hollywood publicists taking a troubled but talented star under their wing, they seem to be intent on promoting autism as a *brand* that just needs better PR. They relentlessly cite movies, Hollywood celebs, and the national attention autism is receiving. It feels almost churlish to focus on autism as injury or disability when there is so much to celebrate and so many galas to attend!

Is there even an epidemic, in their view? "A competing explanation," they say without bothering to assess its dubious merits, "held that the rising numbers throughout the 2000s, rather than marking an epidemic, were a case of epidemiology catching up with reality. In this view, autism, regardless of the specific criteria, was probably always a part of the human condition, but one that it took Leo Kanner to bring into focus, followed by several decades of fine-tuning the definition. It was not that autism was spreading to a larger percentage of the human race than in the past, but that society, prior to 1999, had made no intensive effort to go find the people who were already living with autism among them."[19]

This epidemiological nihilism ends in incoherence. "The lack of evidence of an epidemic was not evidence of *no* epidemic," they continue. Say what now? We are supposed to content ourselves with the idea that there might not *not* be an autism epidemic, or, to turn it around, that one in sixty-eight children might be suffering terribly due to something new in the environment. Or not. How can anyone leave it at that?

Instead, they dwell on rich folks whooping it up for the unfortunates. The book opens with the Night of Too Many Stars gala, where an eleven-year-old blind autistic girl accompanies Katie Perry on the piano for "Firework." "The men were crying too. All around the theater. In the balcony. In the orchestra. On the stage, off to one side, the show's host, Jon Stewart, was seen bringing the back of his hand to his cheek, swiping at it."[20]

Most autism parents cry for different reasons.

Katie Wright, daughter of the founders of Autism Speaks, who saw her son Christian regress after vaccinations, put it this way: "At its very essence regressive autism is about a child losing all the skills and abilities that are necessary to lead a fulfilling independent life. These children lose their speech, gross motor function and even the ability to eat and sleep like normal human beings. Some lucky children regain all the lost skills, but most do not.

"Regressive autism is a catastrophic loss for the child, the child's traumatized family and our country. It costs a lot to have regressive autism. Additionally the majority of these children have epilepsy, serious GI and immune diseases and most remain profoundly disabled all their lives."[21]

Bernard Rimland, the pioneering autism researcher and parent to whom we dedicate this book, wrote to one of us in 2003, ridiculing "the supposedly nonexistent increase in prevalence" of autism. He blasted "the creeps who keep trying to pretend that the autism epidemic is not real." Their "shoddy work in defense of their indefensible theses" should embarrass them and their colleagues, he wrote. "I am reminded of 'Baghdad Bob,' the laughable Minister of Information in Iraq, who continued to defend his indefensible position until he finally disappeared." It was important, Rimland said, to "keep exposing, very professionally, the inadequacy of their work."[22]

That is the mission of this book.

Chapter 1: Desperately Seeking Gulliver traces the history of childhood mental disorders before the first cluster of autism cases was described. In contrast to the claim of "statistical quicksand . . . that made comparisons between past and present exercises in guesswork,"[23] we'll demonstrate that before 1930 childhood mental illness was well-known and extensively documented. Autism was not part of the picture.

Chapter 2: Absence of Evidence: Gulliver in Lilliput looks for broad populations where you would expect to find cases of autism before 1930 if they existed—groups of intellectually disabled and insane children, and records kept by early general practitioners. Here we find almost nothing to suggest autism's presence.

Chapter 3: Evidence of Absence: The Empty Quadrant hunts for case reports of children with mental illness before 1930 that might conceivably be autism. The results are not encouraging for the Epidemic Denial argument.

Chapter 4: Autism Arrives describes the first clusters of autism in the medical literature—in 1943 in Baltimore by Leo Kanner, and in 1944 in Vienna by Hans Asperger. Autism Epidemic Deniers assert this is a coincidence or—even more fancifully—that Kanner took Asperger's discovery and claimed it as his own. In truth, the simultaneous rise points to a common source of causation.

Chapter 5: Unqualified Observers examines the multitude of ways Donvan and Zucker and Silberman misunderstand and misstate the roots and rise of autism, creating an alternative universe that suits their purposes but bears little resemblance to unadorned fact.

Chapter 6: The Epidemic and Its Implications looks at the sharp rise in autism cases in the mid-1990s and the grab bag of excuses, including "better diagnosis," that have been used to deny it, especially the addition of Asperger's to the psychiatrist's bible in the autism category. (Hint: Asperger's is nowhere near enough to account for the twenty-fold rise in diagnoses.)

Chapter 7: The Dynamics of Denial shows how powerful interests have doubled down on suppressing the truth of the epidemic. A modern "mob culture" of bullies has emerged to shout down, shame, and exile anyone who questions the no-epidemic mantra or puts forward a threatening environmental theory.

The Epilogue: Normalizing Autism confronts the real-life consequences of denial. When "the bus stops coming," parents are left to their own devices. When the parents are gone, their adult children become wards of the states. When that happens, the true cost, dimensions, and tragedy of the autism epidemic will be there for all to see. We need to break through this wall of Epidemic Denial *now* to put an end to the worst childhood health crisis in history.

CHAPTER 1

Desperately Seeking Gulliver

"No person can disobey reason, without giving up his claim to be a rational creature."

—Jonathan Swift, *Gulliver's Travels*

◆ ◆ ◆

The child seemed perfectly fine.

Born in 1900 into *fin de siècle* Vienna, a glittering capital of medicine, money and culture, old and new, immigrant and aristocrat, the boy met all the milestones of healthy infancy. He was breast-fed. He smiled. He made eye contact. He pointed. At thirteen months, he began teething. He started walking about the same time, and not long after that he began to talk.

On his third birthday, sometimes described as the transition from infancy to childhood, he was still fine.[24] But the following year, "something changed," according to a doctor who examined him. The intricate, miraculous machinery of human development suddenly sputtered to a stop and shuddered into reverse. The boy became moody. Excitable. Angry. "He cried for hours without provocation. . . . He expressed wishes but nobody could make things right. When he wanted water, the drink that was brought to him was not clean enough. Sometimes he made scenes that lasted for hours.

"Often the boy went to bed and said, 'Mama, I'm sick.' Then he got up after only a few minutes. His food intake was deficient. For months he only ate the same food. He was happy to withdraw from his surroundings." He made rigid movements with his upper body, started stuttering, and "ran around the room" for hours repeating a single word. "He babbled incoherently, hit himself with his hands."

He disappeared in front of their eyes.

Yet the look of intelligent comprehension on his face remained the same, like a car radio obstinately continuing to play upbeat music at the scene of a horrible wreck. Barring injury or some catastrophic illness that left brain damage, this kind of early, complete, permanent mental deterioration was simply unknown to medicine up to that point. So the doctor who examined him hastened to write the case up in a medical journal as the first instance of a new disorder.

In so doing, Wilhelm Weygandt, a German psychiatrist, made a name for himself in the pantheon of medical history. He established "priority" in the naming of a new disorder—his own syndrome.[25]

Gone Boy

The parts of his paper we quote here are, as far as we know, the first time they have appeared in English (translated by our colleague Birgit Calhoun, a native German speaker who works at Stanford Law School's library). That's significant for a number of reasons. Some very important people noticed Weygandt's paper in its original German, most prominently Leo Kanner, discoverer of autism in the 1930s, who said, "More than a quarter-century ago, Weygandt wrote of a number of idiotic and imbecile children who presented schizophrenia-like symptoms. I am quite certain that some of these children must have been typically autistic children." Others have cited Weygandt as among the earliest and strongest evidence that autism had always been around.[26]

But in fact, this was not autism, not the early infantile disorder, not as we now understand it. Many of the symptoms are different, and, crucially, the age of onset was too late. When Kanner first described the disorder that came to be called autism in 1943, he called it *"early infantile autism."* Employing the italics himself, Kanner thought all cases of the strange new disorder were present from birth; he later observed regressions during the first year or two. But it remained a disorder of early infancy, either inborn or in the first twenty-four months of life, emphatically not childhood. In fact, the sentence that begins this chapter—The *child* was perfectly fine—could never be written about a case of autism. The infant and toddler might be fine initially, but the onset of autism symptoms always began before childhood, when the impairment would have been only too obvious.

Not only did autism not exist when Weygandt was describing his own syndrome, there wasn't even a word for it. The word itself was coined in 1911 as *autismus*—a quality of extreme withdrawal and aloneness—by a founder of modern psychiatry, Eugen Bleuler.[27] It came from the Greek root *autos,* meaning self. Bleuler was a pioneering discoverer of schizophrenia, and he coined the term to describe features of schizophrenic withdrawal and introversion. His purpose was narrow; he was describing a trait—not even a dominant one, but helpful in describing the condition. And the need for the description had nothing to do with children.

So the timing and symptoms of Weygandt's patient were significantly different from autism, even though some behaviors—the loss of language, the possibly stereotyped habit of hitting himself with his hands, the running around aimlessly and repeating nonsense phrases—put it in the same ballpark. Notably, the grimacing described by Weygandt and many subsequent observers is not a core feature of autism. And while regression is present in autism, the complete loss of cognitive skills is rare.

The source of the regression puzzled Weygandt. These were children who survived infancy and were developing well. What could have caused it? Casting about, Weygandt speculated about potential injuries—"not-well-known damage to the brain." These children appeared stricken—but by a virus, a toxin, a side effect of medicine, an unrecognized head injury? Weygandt didn't know. (We still don't.)

There seemed no precedent and no category in which to place the unfortunate child. Weygandt published his report in a medical journal devoted to mental illness in the "feeble-minded"—yet this boy had been altogether normal before the regression set in. The journal was devoted to mental retardation and carried the daunting title, *Zeitschrift fur die Erforschung und Behandlung des jugendlichen Schwachsinns.* Modern translation: *Journal for the Study and Treatment of Intellectual Disability.* The article's title was a bit more succinct: *"Idiotie und Dementia Praecox."* Modern Translation: "Intellectual Disability and Schizophrenia."

The article was odd and disjointed. Seven preceding case histories that made up the bulk of Weygandt's paper were all much older than this, Weygandt's final case, and also much different.

A youth identified as IS, for instance, was "a seventeen-year-old feeble-minded girl, [who] reads much in prayer books, goes to church a lot, wants to be a nun. Says she has seen her dead mother. Has worked as a cigar maker. Started to neglect work, laughed for no reason, heard voices, cried, was anxious. Did not eat much but took food away from others. Was institutionalized, thought she needed to pick up the Kaiser. Not much school knowledge. Pulled on her fingers, hopped around the garden. Echolalia. Echopraxia. Typical Hebephrenia."

This is not a foreign language or a mistranslation. The word hebephrenia was part of the language of schizophrenia and described a variety characterized by delusions (needing to pick up the Kaiser), hallucinations (seeing her dead mother), incoherence (repeating back words or mimicking body gestures), and silly behavior (hopping around the garden). The case was typical in developing during the teen years. The other six older cases in the paper were similar; all had intellectual disabilities on top of their mental illnesses.

But what of the four-year-old who disappeared in front of his parents' eyes? Weygandt shoehorned him in, a non sequitur to the thrust of the article, as if getting the child's description into print as quickly as possible was his biggest concern. And in fact, it was. Someone else was on the case—the man who had introduced Weygandt to the four-year-old in the first place. Unlike Weygandt, he had been working on this problem for several years and had already identified a number of children. By rushing the case description into print, Weygandt won the right to claim priority for discovering an exotic and devastating new disorder.

Modern translation: He stole it. Or at least he tried.

◆ ◆ ◆

Weygandt may have announced the disorder to the world first, but priority lay elsewhere. The real discoverer was a Viennese special education teacher named Theodor Heller, who—with his father—ran an institute for handicapped children. Weygandt, a professor in Homberg, accidentally bumped into Heller's investigation in Vienna in 1907. During that visit, Heller asked Weygandt to see the child in question, one of several Heller was observing. Imagine the latter's surprise when the case—and the label *dementia infantilis* that *Heller* had chosen for it—showed up in print under Weygandt's name later that year.

"During his stay in Vienna in 1907," Heller later wrote, "Professor Weygandt had examined psychiatrically one of my cases. I had previously acquainted him with my observations and suggested the name *dementia infantilis* for these cases. Professor Weygandt was able to concur completely with my observations and also accepted the name *dementia infantilis*. This term was chosen merely to designate a state of mental deterioration occurring in childhood."

"Professor Weygandt published the results of these observations during the same year . . . under the title *Idiotie und Dementia Praecox*. Through an oversight the paper fails to refer to my observations and communications."[28] It is clear Heller considered it more than an oversight: he was plainly angry at the breach of professional courtesy. In that same 1930 article, he offered his own account of his work and the process of discovery he clearly believed was his own: "During the years 1905 and 1906 I was given to observe and evaluate an unusually large number of feebleminded children," Heller wrote. "I was particularly impressed by a number of cases in which the past histories were so similar that there could remain no doubt as to a close inner connection. . . . These were children who—without preceding illness—had become conspicuous in their third and fourth years through early symptoms which one might sum up . . . as changes of mood."

These changes affected just about everything: the young child became "disobedient, raging, whining, anxious, sometimes hallucinating," soon lost all language or ability to understand it, "acquired tic-like

5

movements," became incontinent, posed in peculiar positions, needed to be fed. As in many of these cases, his facial contortion described as a grimace caught the observer's attention. The course of the regression was devastating. "Within nine months, the losses were complete and permanent—no improvement was observed in any of the children after that." Heller added in 1930: "The reports about the follow-up studies of children who have gone through a *dementia infantilis* are of interest. All of the children remained in complete idiot regression, did not speak, did not understand anything or only very little."

Like Weygandt, Heller noted the children "maintained their misleading intelligent facial expression," causing parents to be "cruelly disappointed as the low mental status persisted and as the child lapsed into complete idiotic regression." Unlike Weygandt's case series, Heller's cases were closely comparable to one another and markedly different from the classic adult schizophrenia.

Heller's Case 1, TL, was born in Germany in 1891—the earliest birth year of the six children described in his 1908 study and also among the earliest onset. "During her third year of life she began to exhibit angry outbursts without an obvious trigger," Heller reported. "Sometimes she cried for no apparent reason. Later she showed pronounced motor restlessness."

She soiled herself; her language regressed. "Subsequently she exhibited catatonic symptoms (grimacing, salivating, and persisting in fixed gestures, often rolling her eyes outwards and pulling one corner of her mouth inwards)." When Heller first saw her in 1895, "she didn't speak, didn't understand what was said to her and didn't recognize her parents." The outcome? She ended up in an institution with a full-time nurse.

Case 2, KW, was "totally normal into the third year of life," when he became psychotic, talked gibberish, and didn't recognize his parents. As with others, he grimaced and developed tic-like movements.

Case 3 is the four-year-old "boy who was examined by Professor Weygandt in Vienna." Case 4 was strikingly similar, Heller said, a boy whose "speech disappeared but for a few words." He grimaced and played with his fingers. His condition was among the least severe; he could understand directions for simple tasks and enjoyed children's games.

Case 5 was six years old when Heller met him. He was intensely restless, picking up anything on a table, putting it back or throwing it. He had no language but uttered intermittent meaningless sounds. Case 6, from Turkey, regressed in his fourth year with "irritability and aversion to any activity," anger, sudden agitation, loss of language—a by-now familiar pattern to Heller. "There is no spontaneity. The boy requires constant observation. If he is alone, he makes windmilling movements with the upper part of his body. He swings and spins his arms and hands. His sleep is sufficient and uninterrupted now."

In all the cases Heller observed, "a misleading appearance of intelligent facial expression is noticeable, despite the deep level of dementia." Like Weygandt, he grappled with the question of *why* the children had deteriorated so suddenly and at such a consistent point in childhood. What were the possible causes? One had a wet nurse that had been "successfully" treated for syphilis, probably with mercury; another regressed at the same time his family moved; a third had a fall; a fourth had her adenoids removed. Some had slight developmental delays or "a minor degree of intellectual disability before their regression," but not enough to explain what ultimately happened, nor to account for a cluster of several such children in one place where none had been reported before.

Heller took pains to distinguish his syndrome from conventional intellectual disability (the condition that went by the then-current "idiocy"). "*Dementia infantilis* is characterized by a period of normal or almost normal mental development," Heller emphasized. "None of the explanations given for the changes sufficiently account for the rapid mental regression."[29]

More than Weygandt, Heller became the acknowledged expert, the go-to clinician for this novel disorder. He saw numerous cases over the coming years, the most of any single author. Even so, his roster of patients never became very large. By the time he wrote his 1930 follow-up, he had "collected" just twenty-eight cases in a quarter century, barely one per year.

The Gulliver Paradox

Let's pause here on this seemingly obscure episode in medical history to connect it to the issue of autism. The Epidemic Denial theory—that autism hasn't really increased at all—requires centuries of observational failure in the medical and educational professionals who cared for children. In stark contrast to the presumption of negligence in overlooking autism stand Wilhelm Weygandt and Theodor Heller. When Heller and subsequently Weygandt saw the four-year-old boy in 1907, they immediately recognized his condition was new and noteworthy. For his part, Heller knew he wanted a doctor to look at one of these children; as for the doctor, after observing the child, Weygandt ran, not walked, to the nearest medical journal to share the joy (and prestige) of his discovery. While Heller was carefully assembling his findings, Professor Weygandt (perhaps more greedy for the spoils of academic acclaim) shoehorned his novel finding into an account he had nearly completed about intellectually disabled teenagers.

If you're an Autism Epidemic Denier, you're going to have a hard time with what today is called Heller's, Heller-Weygandt syndrome, or Childhood Disintegrative Disorder (CDD). The reason has to do with the relative frequency of each condition and the utter fatuity of claiming the far more common one (autism) could be missed while its fantastically rare older cousin (Heller-Weygandt, now CDD) could be documented, fought over, and followed for decades before the first notice of autism in 1943. Heller's is as rare now as when the educator first assembled his list of cases, around one in fifty thousand children. By contrast, today's autism rate is one in sixty-eight, three orders of magnitude—one thousand times—more common.

The Heller-Weygandt saga demonstrates clearly that medical and education professionals were on the job by the early twentieth century, fully capable of recognizing, describing, coveting credit for, and publicizing a distinctive condition of early childhood. The Deniers reject even that possibility. They need to believe—they need *you* to believe—that autism was somehow missed all along and what is now taking place is an epidemic of recognition rather than cases. That's an extraordinary claim, and extraordinary claims require extraordinary proof. If they were right, Deniers would need to demonstrate a pattern of carelessness in medical history, failure to observe mental illness in children in rigorous ways, and mislabeling of children who today would be clearly diagnosed as autistic.

The Heller-Weygandt saga dramatically illustrates the falsity of the argument that autism was always around yet somehow unobserved. The condition Heller and Weygandt described was clear; it was clearly not autism; it was rare; and it was observed rigorously and by numerous researchers. How would it be possible for autism to exist alongside the observations of Heller, Weygandt, and dozens of others, yet go unnoticed? This alleged negligence, which makes no logical, real-world sense whatsoever, is central to the Denier arguments.

We call this the Gulliver Deception, with autism in the role of Gulliver. Like the relative giant roaming among the tiny Lilliputians in Jonathan Swift's *Gulliver's Travels*, autism towers in scale and significance above other concerns and disabling conditions of childhood. The social toll is enormous, its cost will be crippling, and it dwarfs the scale of disorders like Heller-Weygandt.

That's where Deniers are cornered by their own argument—there is just no hiding their supposed ever-present, but previously overlooked or misdiagnosed, horde of autistic children behind adjacent childhood conditions like Heller-Weygandt. There simply isn't room. Yet Deniers live in a world in which the occasional glint of an autistic trait in some historical figure propels their narrative toward heroic heights based on evidence-free claims of constant prevalence. The absence of actual compelling case descriptions or broader reports of affected populations simply doesn't matter to them. They use documentation of cases like Heller's and Weygandt's to create fog and uncertainty around their theory of recognition. They fail to ask tough questions such as the following: if child psychiatrists in the early twentieth century could observe, describe, and define a condition like Heller-Weygandt, how could they have missed a far more common and equally vivid condition like autism?

We've learned in our research that Heller and Weygandt weren't alone. Dozens of others confirmed the phenomenon that Heller labeled *dementia infantilis*. Some even came up with other names like *dementia praecocissima,* But Heller's label and thorough description attracted the most supporters. These supports came from all over the world.

One of the most prominent was Julius Zappert, like Heller a Viennese, but unlike him a doctor and researcher whose work over many decades ran the gamut from post-vaccine brain injury to early reports of polio. He wrote learned chapters in authoritative medical volumes, chapters such as "Organic Diseases of the Nervous System" for the text *The Diseases of Children—a Work for the Practicing Physician,* a contribution first published in English in 1908, the year Heller's own report appeared. Later, Heller wrote with approval of Zappert's synthesis of the criteria for differential diagnosis:

> Various authors have since described cases of *dementia infantilis* (Higier, Jancke, and others). More recently in 1921, Julius Zappert made *dementia infantilis* the topic for a presentation at the meeting of the German Pediatric Association . . . at Jena. His material comprised thirteen cases, in all of whom he could consistently observe the following stages:
>
> 1. Normal mental and physical development during the first years of life;
> 2. Onset of the illness between the third and fourth years of life;
> 3. Psychic and intellectual changes demonstrated by ineffectiveness of educational and recreational . . . influences; marked restlessness, excited and occasionally anxious behavior, increasing dementia;
> 4. Appearance of speech disorders in the beginning and during the course of the illness;
> 5. Maintenance of motor functions and complete lack of focal symptoms from the central nervous system;
> 6. Final complete idiotic regression;
> 7. Non-imbecile facial expression and looks ('Blick.').

◆ ◆ ◆

So there was plenty of confirmation that Heller and Weygandt had recognized and diagnosed a rare new disorder that showed up from time to time in other clinics throughout Europe. It was defined in some respects by its onset in the third or fourth year of life—practically speaking, between two and a half and four years of age. It had a distinctive cluster of symptoms, most tragically marked by a near complete loss of cognitive function that was permanent. Despite that, the strikingly intelligent appearance, one that distinguished it from conventional idiocy, led parents fruitlessly to seek a cure from doctors and psychiatrists. The disorder was observed and confirmed multiple times by numerous researchers including Leo Kanner, who eventually was the first to describe autism: All of them remarked on its consistent and striking features, and all of them remarked that it was rare. In short, it was distinctive in the way autism was distinctive. And the story of its emergence and discovery provides compelling evidence against the better-diagnosing theory of autism. If autism had been there, these diagnosticians would have found it, too. And they would have found it hundreds of times more often.

But let's not claim too much with this one episode. Heller-Weygandt isn't the only disabling condition of early childhood that plausibly shares autistic traits. Childhood schizophrenia, in which *autismus* or self-absorption to the exclusion of the real world is a characteristic trait, was also observed, and it is to these children we turn next.

Madness is Hard to Miss

Insanity. Madness. Psychosis. *Dementia praecox.* Schizophrenia. Hebephrenia. Whatever label we use, severe mental illness is frightening, dramatic, ruinous, occasionally comic, potentially fatal to self and others and—inevitably—inherently interesting. Literature is full of vivid, sometimes lurid, sometimes laughable descriptions of demented characters, from Jack Nicholson's violently psychotic "Here's Johnny!" to John Nash's "Beautiful Mind." The fact that around 1 percent of the population develops schizophrenia—initially termed *dementia praecox*—has been known since the industrial revolution. Like *dementia infantilis, dementia praecox* was marked by the deterioration from a previously normal mental state. In the case of *dementia praecox,* that regression typically occurred in adolescence and early adulthood.

Numerous observers described the symptoms of madness, from John Haslam at Bethlem Asylum to Henry Maudsley in his landmark discussion of insanity, "The Physiology and Pathology of the Mind." Emil Kraepelin, in Germany, brought diagnostic clarity to the field in the late 1800s, broadly classifying mental disorders (the undifferentiated miasma of "madness") into two predominant types—affective and psychotic. The former—affective means emotional—were mostly depression (then called melancholy) and mania (now bipolar). The latter type, psychosis, was characterized by hallucinations and delusions; Kraepelin labeled the descent into madness *dementia praecox,* nodding to the fact that the loss of mental skills—dementia—could be a familiar feature of old age like senility, but that mental disintegration in adolescence was horribly premature.

In recent decades, Kraepelin's original division has been sliced and diced many times, with no truly stable diagnostic framework. Depression has been expanded; schizophrenia has been declared a spectrum (but no longer paranoid); bipolar and schizoaffective disorder describe other varieties and blends of madness.

While his terminology has not survived, Kraepelin receives widespread recognition for his contributions to systematizing descriptions of mental illness. His pioneering work in the nineteenth century provides another rebuttal to Denier theories, because any disorder as vivid and frequent as autism would surely have found its way into the medical canon of careful observers like Kraepelin, whose renown was worldwide and whose work ran to thousands of pages before 1900.

In 1911, Eugene Bleuler, the German psychiatrist who coined the term *autismus,* revamped Kraepelin's diagnostic categories and coined the word *schizophrenia* for psychotic disorders that begin in adolescence or early adulthood. For a while, the two systems competed, so you'll see *dementia praecox* used into the 1930s in the United States, usually interchangeably with schizophrenia; one of Leo Kanner's mentors at Johns Hopkins, Adolf Meyer, did much to popularize the American understanding of *dementia praecox.*

In our search for Gulliver—the supposed hidden horde with ever-present autism throughout history—it's important to note that schizophrenia was also observed in children. And while in most cases the onset was ten years of age or later, there were scattered reports of schizophrenia in younger children. These reports were controversial; some even doubted the existence of schizophrenia with an onset before ten. But if the Deniers couldn't unmask Gulliver disguised as Heller-Weygandt syndrome, perhaps childhood schizophrenia offered another means of concealment?

That's a problem. As with Heller-Weygandt, most observers consider childhood schizophrenia to be extremely rare. Not a promising place for

Gulliver to hide. Before he saw his first case of autism in 1938, Leo Kanner wrote about childhood schizophrenia in his 1935 textbook. "Parergastic [psychotic] reactions are very infrequently seen to develop before the age of puberty. But such cases undoubtedly exist." Kanner didn't claim personal knowledge of such cases but cited the experience of a researcher named Theodor Ziehen: "In extremely rare instances he could trace the development of typical schizophrenia back to the seventh year of life."

The *seventh* year of life! This is dramatically later than the Heller-Weygandt cases, which came on in the third or fourth year. Ziehen here pegs the earliest onset of schizophrenia to the seventh year, even further away from autism. Childhood schizophrenia cases like Ziehen's are bumping up against the boundary of precocious puberty; if puberty provides the biological stimulation for schizophrenia's onset, perhaps the same mechanisms could be at work in some cases of "childhood schizophrenia."

◆ ◆ ◆

As we've scoured the literature on childhood mental illness in the nineteenth and early twentieth centuries, we've looked hard for reports of childhood schizophrenia. Like Kanner, we found such reports to be extremely rare, with cases of early onset schizophrenia much harder to find than Heller-Weygandt. Numerous authors commented on the rarity of childhood schizophrenia; nevertheless, a few provided case descriptions that support its existence. One of the earliest of these reports came from Howard Potter, former assistant director of the New York State Psychiatric Institute and Hospital. In 1932, Potter reported six cases of early onset schizophrenia, with the earliest possible onset coming at three and a half years of age. This was an odd case, one that matches no established criteria. Nevertheless, Potter concluded "that the child has had clinical schizophrenia since the onset of the first attack at the age of 3.5 years," as well as a current attack of schizophrenia-type symptoms that recurred when he was ten years old.

In a lengthy review paper, "Schizophrenia In Children," that he read at the American Psychiatric Association meeting in Philadelphia in 1932, Potter described his six cases while also surveying the field of schizophrenia in children in general. He combined a reflection on the nature of children's mental disorders with a definition of schizophrenia that he could apply to children. He discussed observations from around the world of early onset cases of schizophrenia, commenting that "psychodynamically, regression is a characteristic of schizophrenia in children as well as in adults." Once again, the later regression that characterizes schizophrenia stands in stark contrast to the first autism cases that would emerge subsequently in that same decade. Potter noted the different way schizophrenia might manifest itself in childhood, since children lack the relationships and experience to create florid psychoses. "Delusional formations seen in childhood are relatively simple and their symbolization is particularly naïve," Potter said.

Following Potter, Mildred Creak made a similar set of observations in 1937. In her paper "Psychoses in Children," Creak reviewed the literature and described thirty-five cases. "The onset of definite symptoms . . . in all but nine, lay between the ages of 13 and 15. These nine cases were of earlier onset." How much earlier she left unspecified but there is no suggestion that they were as early as Heller-Weygandt cases and certainly not evident in infancy. One case out of the nine "had an indefinite onset when she was about seven years old."

In 1938, the same year Leo Kanner saw the first child with autism in Baltimore, an extensive literature review of "Schizophrenia-Like Psychoses in Young Children" provided a valuable retrospective; we have found no more comprehensive treatment. (It's one that Deniers like Silberman and Donvan and Zucker omit entirely.) R. A. Q. Lay, a physician at Guy's Hospital in London, condensed the findings of dozens of medical papers from all over the world including German, Italian, French, and English contributions. He emphatically confirms the point we have been demonstrating here: when it came to mental illness in children, there were two Rs—regressive and rare.

First, regression. "Common to all are regressive changes leading especially to loss of recent attainments, and to some disorganization of the personality following a hitherto normal development," Lay wrote. Note the phrase—regression was "common to all." *All*. When we peg the rate of autism (which was never regressive in its early manifestations) before this moment as effectively zero, we are simply following the lead of the best and most comprehensive body of work to that point. It may seem counterintuitive, but it is not counterfactual.

14

Second, rarity. Lay itemized rarity by pointing to studies like Strecker's in the *New York Medical Journal* in 1927; he was able to find only eighteen cases of psychosis in children among five thousand admissions to a Philadelphia hospital; of these, four were *dementia praecox*, ten manic-depressive, and four of doubtful type. All, however, were over ten years of age at the onset.

So it went down the list of studies and observations: Emil Kraepelin, the great systematizer of psychiatry, wrote in 1913 that of 1,054 cases of schizophrenia he had observed, just 3.5 percent developed before the age of ten. And as we've seen elsewhere, that mostly meant ages seven, eight, and nine—not from infancy, and certainly not from birth. Lay cited numerous reports of low rates of schizophrenia in childhood: "The rarity of psychoses in children is especially commented on prior to 1914. In this year, Rhein published a paper in which he had collected 44 cases under 16 years of age from the literature. But of these only 2 were under 15 among 5,000 consecutive hospital admissions." (After 1914, Heller-Weygandt began to emerge.)

Lay reported not just prevalence rates but also provided an extensive catalog of such reports. His review describes dozens of reports including both childhood schizophrenia and *dementia infantilis*. In addition to his literature review, Lay also reported a case series of six children. Of these, the prevailing diagnoses were Heller-Weygandt syndrome, but he also commented on the importance of differentiating between that, childhood schizophrenia, and even encephalitis leading to mental deterioration. None of his cases were, to his mind, clear-cut examples of early onset schizophrenia.

If you're an Autism Epidemic Denier, you're going to have as hard a time dealing with childhood schizophrenia as with Heller-Weygandt. It once again highlights the rarity of childhood mental illness of any kind and the complete absence of ones with onset from birth or infancy. Gulliver certainly can't be hiding here.

Starting in 1938, the landscape of these case reports began to change, especially in the United States.

Writing in the same year as Lay, Louise Despert's "Schizophrenia in Children" foreshadowed a change in the balance of childhood mental disorders. Despert wrote "schizophrenia in children is not so rare as has long been thought" and described twenty-nine cases admitted to the

New York State Psychiatric Institute between 1930 and 1937. Eighteen of her cases had onset before seven years of age. But none of them are described individually. It's quite possible she was beginning to see cases in New York similar to Leo Kanner's in Baltimore during that period. If she did see a case that qualified as autistic, however, she didn't find it notable enough to report. The one case she describes in detail appears to match Heller-Weygandt syndrome, although she doesn't call it that.

By 1947, four years after Kanner's landmark article, Lauretta Bender described a landscape of childhood mental illness that had begun to shift markedly. In her paper "Childhood Schizophrenia," Bender provided "a clinical study of 100 schizophrenic children." In this case population, Bender described three groups, one that clearly matched Heller-Weygandt syndrome, another that matched childhood schizophrenia, but a third that comprised an earlier onset group with symptoms similar to what Kanner was reporting as autism. In fact, Despert referred directly to Kanner's report. "The youngest schizophrenic children," she wrote, "those in the first two or three years of life, showed disturbances in the vegetative rhythms and habit patterns, in motility, and in object relationship. Mothers are most distressed by this inability of the child to relate to herself, to siblings, play material, food or clothes. Language has no objective use for sign value, communication or interpersonal relations. Kanner speaks of 'autistic disturbances in affective contact.'"

This description of her new group is clearly, and suddenly, autism—recall how long we have been looking for children with onset at age two or below. Just as clearly, these cases described by Kanner and Bender could have been observed decades earlier by observers like Heller and Weygandt *had they been there to see.* This argues against the notion, often expressed, that it took a clinician of Kanner's observational powers (and they were considerable) to spot something like autism and tease it out from its companion disorders. No, what it took were the first cases actually occurring.

Bender describes a second group she distinguishes from the earliest onset cases. Again, precision in defining the age of onset is crucial. "From three to four and a half years is the most common period of onset. . . . In six months the child may lose all he has gained in three years, especially the socially oriented behavior patterns, leaving him well developed physically with good gait and exaggerated graceful motility, but having lost many of his acquired habit patterns, language, object relationship, with increased anxiety and physical dependence on the mother." Bender clearly places this group within a known diagnostic category. "Regressive mental illnesses or infantile dementia commonly starting at this age have been recognized for some time as Heller's Disease."

Finally, Bender's taxonomy includes a third group, which is clearly recognizable as childhood schizophrenia. She places the onset of these cases as prepubertal, starting at the age of ten to eleven and one half. Notably, she considers and rejects the notion of childhood schizophrenia emerging before ten years of age. Instead, she considers reports of early onset childhood schizophrenia to be overlooked cases of Heller's disease. "Children of school age are often brought to the psychiatrists' attention with a history of onset apparently at 6 to 8 years. In most of these, however, it is probable that the onset was three to four years and only recognized when the child was brought to school and into community activities." Setting aside Bender's presumption of the underdiagnosis of Heller's disease, her rejection of the possibility of early onset childhood schizophrenia speaks to the rarity of the condition.

So was childhood schizophrenia a cloak hiding Gulliver? Clearly not. Numerous authors wrote about childhood schizophrenia, and all of them distinguished Heller-Weygandt syndrome from other instances of regressive disorders. Before 1940, there were no observations of any condition with an onset preceding Heller's. As far as cases with later onset, schizophrenia was seen to emerge in childhood, but cases before ten years of age were extremely rare. For observers like Bender, the sudden arrival of early onset cases directed unprecedented attention to the lower border of childhood—the third birthday—and, more importantly, the time preceding it. For everyone until Bender and Kanner, that early period had been virtually devoid of observable mental illness.

Brains on Fire

Core features that define all these separate diagnostic frameworks are both the nature (regressive or not) and timing of onset (the age at which the symptoms are visible). More than individual symptoms, which may or may not have an underlying biological reality, a deep physiological divide separates different stages of brain development. The growth rate of the human brain is both extraordinary and variable during the early years of life.

We wrote about this in *The Age of Autism*. "In an evolutionary sense, a large brain is the organ that has made humans exceptional animals. A long journey of natural selection separated primates from the rest of the placental mammals, then separated the genus Homo from apes and ultimately left Homo sapiens the sole survivor among the genus: the world's only upright-walking, symbolic-thinking, language-speaking species. Most of that journey was marked by the increasing size of our most exceptional organ, our brains. Just as the large relative size of the primate brain is the key trait that distinguishes primates from other mammals, similarly, the large relative size of the human brain is the key trait that distinguishes humans from other primates. In adult humans (based on typical primate development models), the brain is bigger by about four times than it should be given our size."

Humans and other advanced primates such as chimpanzees are born with big brains. It might be surprising to some, but most of the divergence in human and primate brain size comes after birth, when the human brain is undergoing the greatest changes in the entire life span. The rate of brain growth in an infant is nothing short of explosive. Before thirty months, every spare ounce of energy an infant's body can generate is directed toward that growth process. After three years of age, everything settles down; by six years of age a boy's brain is as large as his mother's, and by ten years of age any child's brain is just about fully grown. The chart below demonstrates this dynamic: whether you are measuring brain growth by absolute weight or percentage growth, there is no comparable human developmental window beyond the first thirty-month (thirty-nine if you include in utero) biological process in human life.

The changes in the human brain while it's undergoing this explosive growth are too numerous to contemplate. As tissue expands, neurons are formed and migrate, connections are made and pruned, cells differentiate and specialize. Meanwhile, external inputs interact with the physical capabilities of the brain, as a child's acquisition of skills is

18

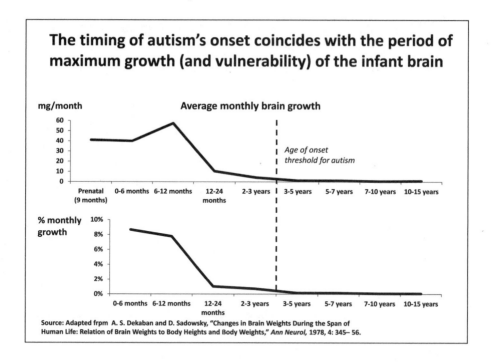

The timing of autism's onset coincides with the period of maximum growth (and vulnerability) of the infant brain

Source: Adapted frpm A. S. Dekaban and D. Sadowsky, "Changes in Brain Weights During the Span of Human Life: Relation of Brain Weights to Body Heights and Body Weights," *Ann Neurol*, 1978, 4: 345– 56.

critically related to how the brain processes those inputs during crucial developmental windows. It's remarkable how many of these complex developments take place without going haywire, but when something does go wrong, the consequences are usually irreversible.

Autism's onset during this window is what makes it unique, and autism's unique impairments—of language, socialization, novelty seeking—all reflect disruptions of normal brain development. What's truncated or diverted in unproductive ways are developmental skills that emerge in that early window—a baby's first words, the recognition of other humans and the connection with them, and the initial exploration (crawling, walking, touching, tasting of the outside world). One tragedy of autism lies in the way it interferes with developing the key elements that define our humanity. As we wrote in *The Age of Autism*: "Humans are particularly social, yet autism selectively disables the capacity for 'affective contact.' We are novelty seekers, we make tools, explore the globe, and invent new technologies; but autism brutally restricts the interests of the affected." We are the only species on the planet with language, yet autism attacks that capability too, sometimes destroying it. "In a sense, as we search for the roots of autism we are seeking out the distinctive biology of the human experience."

So in the search for a differential diagnosis of any childhood mental disorder, nothing matters more than timing of onset. This shouldn't be surprising. Any parent knows the mental state of a walking, talking three-year-old toddler is light years away from an infant of a year and a half—for one thing, they're twice as old. When we observe marked distinctions in symptom clusters among mental disorders, we ignore age of onset at our peril. But in the world of the Deniers there is no special significance to minor details like this. Everyone with a disability is all a part of the great neurodiversity tribe. It makes no difference when you join.

◆ ◆ ◆

We believe the clear identification of Heller's and childhood schizophrenia by the first decade of the twentieth century, without a commensurate recognition of a much more common disorder we now call autism, demolishes Epidemic Denial at its foundations. As Swift put it, if you disobey reason, you are not a rational creature.

CHAPTER 2

Absence of Evidence:
Gulliver in Lilliput

"Yesterday, upon the stair,
I met a man who wasn't there.
He wasn't there again today,
I wish, I wish he'd go away."
—From "Antigonish" by William Hughes Mearns, 1899

We've seen that a disease that affects 1.5 percent of children is not easily hidden in known disorders like Heller-Weygandt and childhood schizophrenia. Both were exceedingly rare, readily observable, widely described, and clearly not autism. So if our search for Gulliver were defined by looking for autism disguised as (or behind) other well-defined syndromes, it seems blindingly obvious that the rate of autism was effectively zero before 1930.

Or was it? Perhaps we are being unnecessarily narrow in refining our search to a world of known disorders like Heller-Weygandt and childhood schizophrenia. Perhaps there are other ways to search for the Gulliver of autism. Instead of looking bottom-up, an alternative approach is to look instead in a more top-down fashion, identifying broader populations in which large groups of people we have known through history have been disabled.

There are at least three population types that we can explore, populations that are rich with sources containing early descriptions of children, sources where one would reasonably expect to find Gulliver if there was an autism rate of one in sixty-eight at any given time. These three populations include the following:

- Intellectually disabled children. The nomenclature for these populations has changed with time, with scientific fashion, with compassion/political correctness. Observers of this population have variously defined the category as made up of idiots, imbeciles, aments, the mentally retarded, and so on. As far as our hunt for autism goes, the people in this population are almost always affected by mental incapacity from birth, so age of onset would be less of an issue. If Gulliver were hiding here, descriptions of this group should be rich with autism cases and autism-like symptoms.

- Mad or insane populations. Within such populations there might be references to early onset "insanity," which on closer inspection match the profile of autism. We've seen that childhood schizophrenia is an unrewarding place to search for Gulliver, but within groups of insane people variously described as mad, psychotic, and schizophrenic, perhaps we'll find descriptions that match the profile of autism. Until recently, this population was easy to locate—in madhouses, asylums, and state hospitals.

- Community doctors' patient populations. Before we entered the age of legislated privacy and electronic medical records, where physicians practice out of groups and hospitals in a transactional manner, doctors worked in a much more intimate setting with their patients. A single doctor would often cover an entire community and as a routine part of the practice take extensive notes on each individual patient. One such doctor's notes have been used for detailed analysis of health profiles of residents of seventeenth century England, including, fortuitously, children.

Let's take a look at each of these populations in depth through a selection of the best-known publications that describe them.

Intellectually Disabled Populations

The idea that mental retardation shielded what we now call autism seems at first glance to make a lot of sense. It is perhaps the most powerful of the Denier arguments, persisting even today in the claim of diagnostic substitution—that autism is simply replacing mental disability in school-based education services, in some cases because parents "want" the diagnosis to result in better services for their kids, or because it sounds more respectable or hopeful than some form of intelligence deficit. We mentioned this alleged "substitution" of one diagnosis for another in the introduction and will come back to current data on that question later.

A full review of the medical literature on mental retardation would take more space than we have here. But there are several comprehensive accounts, some of which have already played a role in the autism debate; these provide a rich opportunity to look for Gulliver decades and even centuries before Kanner's 1943 paper describing the first case series.

In 1848, Samuel Gridley Howe conducted a comprehensive survey—"the Condition of the Idiots of the Commonwealth" of Massachusetts."[30] In 1867, John Langdon Down wrote a famous paper "on the ethnic classification of idiots," where he described what we now call Down syndrome. Over the next twenty years, he continued to work with intellectual disability and in 1887 published a broader collection of observations titled *On Some of the Mental Affections of Childhood and Youth.*[31] Following Down in 1898, William W. Ireland's *On Idiocy and Imbecility,* a four-hundred-forty-page compendium, included observations "on insanity in children and insane idiots."[32] In 1908, Alfred Frank Tredgold went further than Ireland, writing over five hundred pages on *Mental Deficiency,* subtitled *Amentia.*[33] Like Ireland, Tredgold also wrote about the overlap of insanity and intellectual disability, including in his book a chapter on "Insane Aments."

◆ ◆ ◆

That last category, despite its hopelessly dated terminology, is a good starting point because the likeliest hiding place for autism among the mentally disabled would be those who also suffered from insanity. Tredgold writes:

A large number of aments react to their environment in a perfectly consistent, uniform, and as far as their mental capacity will admit, normal manner, and such may be considered sane, albeit defective. On the other hand, a certain number are characterized by lapses from their ordinary mental state of such intensity that, for the time being, they may be rightly termed insane; it is with these latter that this chapter deals.

So what is that "certain number" of intellectually disabled people—aments—who are also mentally ill—insane? Tredgold offers a surprisingly precise answer. He estimated that about 8 percent, or 4,450 people out of "the total feeble-minded of the country (54,114)," were what he termed "feeble-minded insane."[34] Notice that's a far bigger number than the few dozen cases Heller began cataloging that same year. There's more room for Gulliver here, but still not enough. Given the population of England at the time, 40.175 million, there should have been 591,000 people with autism, 132 times more than the 4,450 "feeble-minded insane" among whom we are looking for even one possibly misdiagnosed case of autism. Even if all cognitively disabled people in Britain in 1908 had autism, all 54,114 of them, we'd still be less than a tenth of the way to the current autism rate. But maybe enough scattered cases were in Tredgold's account to give some glint of Gulliver's presence, some ray of hope for the Deniers whose entire argument rests on their presence? Sadly (for them), no.

Tredgold writes that mentally disabled children who go on to develop insanity show "instability" such as "fits of irritability, moroseness or bad temper, [and] although these conditions can hardly be termed insanity, they are the shadows of the coming event. In the majority of cases, however, the first attack makes its appearance between the periods of puberty and adolescence, and in some cases even much earlier than this."[35] Puberty and adolescence is the time frame for the onset of schizophrenia, and it shouldn't be surprising that a percentage of the intellectually disabled, just like a percentage of the rest of the population, succumbs to it. This sounds very similar to the group Weygandt wrote about in his 1907 paper—a case series about teenagers and young adults with intellectual impairment developing severe mental illness.

As for the "much earlier" cases that Tredgold describes, his case histories make clear he is not talking about infants, as would by definition be the case with autism. Intellectual disability, barring some accident or illness that came later, was always present from birth or evident in infancy; mental illness, it seems, almost never was. To take the first of the cases Tredgold offers to "illustrate this type of mentally unstable aments," consider Thomas B., "a feeble-minded young man, twenty-five years of age, with numerous stigmata of degeneracy. He could never learn at school, and afterwards could not keep his situations. At the age of 23 he became insane, and was sent to the asylum for six months."

On through the standard mental illnesses the case histories went, from mania to melancholia to stupor to delusional insanity, none sounding like autism or described as present from birth or early infancy. Instead, they followed the trajectory of Thomas B.:

- MD, female. "At the age of 19 years she began to get mischievous and destructive, and finally became so troublesome that she had to be sent to an asylum."
- TC, male. "At 15 years of age he began to get very bad-tempered and strange in his manner; he had attacks of screaming, which lasted for hours; and ultimately, at 17 years, was sent to an asylum with acute mania."

So the Gulliver of autism was certainly not hidden among Tredgold's patients. If they existed in any material numbers, Tredgold would have been a good place for them to start showing themselves. It is, of course, possible that a case of what we would now call autism is embedded among the thousands of cases of intellectual disability Tredgold (and others) cite. But the fact that until 1943 none were identified as in any way different from others is highly significant—the absence of evidence with which this chapter is concerned.

Kanner said in his 1943 paper that most of his eleven cases "were at one time or another looked upon as feeble-minded," but that on further inspection the diagnosis did not hold up. "They are all unquestionably endowed with good *cognitive potentialities*," he wrote, emphasizing the cognitive part with italics. And they all bore "strikingly intelligent physiognomies," which further reduces the pool of autistics conceivably misdiagnosed in this way in the past. The Kanner associate who first saw Virginia S., the eldest child in his case series, in a "state training school for the feeble-minded" remarked in a phrase that ought to be etched on the tombstone of the Denier argument that "Virginia stands out from other children because she is absolutely different. . . . "[36]

To repopulate the world pre-1930 with hundreds of thousands of autistic people such as Virginia S., and claim they were misdiagnosed as mentally disabled, you'd need to isolate the ones who look "strikingly intelligent"—a very small proportion—with good cognitive potential, whose behavior in infancy showed signs not just of mental impairment but of autism. Given the fact that 31.6 percent of children with autism today have a co-diagnosis of intellectual disability (IQ of seventy or below), many such cases should have been evident in Tredgold's population. There were not.

◆ ◆ ◆

Still, let's keep looking. Moving backward in time, William Wotherspoon Ireland looked at the category of mental illness within the broader population of mentally challenged children he was studying. In 1898 in England, he published *On Idiocy and Imbecility,*[37] two words for low IQ. In 1890, he calculated the "number of idiots" was 95,571. That translates to 1.5 percent—or just about the same rate as autism today. Thus, as we saw with Tredgold, if autism were hiding behind mental deficiency, a significant percentage of the latter should also have had clear signs of the former.

In a chapter titled "On Insanity in Children and Insane Idiots and Imbeciles," Ireland notes "insanity in children is a rare affliction" and generally connected with illness like meningitis, and that the most frequent forms are mania and melancholy. He describes a girl of six admitted to an asylum suffering from mania, convulsions, and an inability to speak. Another, a boy of thirteen described as "a dull child," had been "so often punished at school, on account of his slow progress, that he became deeply melancholy, and tried to kill himself."[38] The melancholy alternated with mania, suggesting a bipolar condition that may or may not have been triggered by the way he was treated.

Younger children were also affected, but not young enough to be considered autistic. "Great fretfulness, striking, biting, and destructiveness, which are occasionally observed in children from three to four years of age . . . are to be regarded as true mania." Ireland cites another case of a girl of five who had "been quite healthy up to the fourth year of life," followed by intermittent fever and whooping cough that lasted fourteen weeks and was severe enough to cause nosebleeds. "Soon after, the first symptoms of mental derangement were observed," including hallucinations and the delusion that her food "contained injurious substances." This is quite clearly a post pertussis encephalitis. She subsequently died.

Another girl was healthy into her third year when she began having symptoms of epilepsy. "She became very mischievous, tearing her clothes, stabbing her horse with a knife, and attacking children." At twelve, she tried to set her father's house on fire and put out her aunt's children's eyes with a hairpin. An autopsy showed severe brain abnormalities no doubt related to the epilepsy and, almost certainly, to her behavior. Other cases point to biological causes as well, including a child who had encephalitis at eight months: "I have seen a case of insanity in a girl aged eleven, where the most prominent features are great oddity of expression, and complaints of having been subjected to ill usage, which seem to be delusions. She takes severe epileptic fits."

So Ireland saw plenty of insanity in children, but none whose age or affliction bring autism to mind.

Ireland coined the term "genetous idiocy," in which the "deficient mental manifestation is complete before birth and the presumption of a hereditary condition is stronger than in other forms." Often it runs in the family—"there are often parents, aunts, or uncles who have been insane, imbecilic, epileptic or deaf, or have suffered from some other disorder of the nervous system."

Just as psychiatry had terms like hebephrenia, schizophrenia, catatonia and so on, the study of mental deficiency had many categories. Besides genetous idiocy, Ireland listed eleven more[39]:

1. Genetous idiocy

27

2. Microcephalic idiocy
3. Hydrocephaic idiocy
4. Eclampsic idiocy
5. Epileptic idiocy
6. Paralytic idiocy
7. Traumatic idiocy
8. Inflammatory idiocy (the result of encephalitis)
9. Sclerotic idiocy
10. Syphilitic idiocy
11. Cretinism
12. Idiocy by deprivation

While we might use different terms here, the thing to notice is that each of the categories is assigned a cause, such as inflammatory idiocy that might be caused by an illness, or syphilis in which the condition passes from the mother at birth. Head injuries and "deprivation," presumably lack of proper feeding, is another. In effect, only the first one hides its roots in the genes but shows itself in a family tendency toward the disorder.

Once again, contrast this with autism. None of the injuries or illnesses during or after birth has been associated in any significant way with autism. Even the genetous category is inadequate because, while some children with autism appear different from birth, they seldom have any significant number of close relatives who also have autism. In fact, a common observation among parents is that no one in their extended families has ever had a condition like this. Nor is it possible after birth to link regressive autism to a particular event such as an accident or severe illness; that may cause brain damage—Tredgold's amentia—but not the characteristic behaviors of autism.

◆ ◆ ◆

Tredgold's and Ireland's treatments are similar, but also obscure. By contrast, many who claim autism is ancient rest their case on the work of John Haydon Langdon Down, the century's premier diagnostician of mental disorders. His most enduring discovery was Down Syndrome, which he wrote about in 1866 in a paper title "Observations on an ethnic classification of idiots,"[40] since those with three copies of chromosome 21—a "trisomy 21"—bore an Asiatic look. Twenty-one years later he published a broader series of lectures based on "nearly 30 years of observation in London," probably of children born from the late 1850s to 1885.

Here is where Down's observations include some children with what might be described as autistic features. Along with Down syndrome and other categories of intellectual disability, he described two smaller groups—a "developmental" one and an "accidental" one—that researchers like Darold A. Treffert, MD, have argued correspond to regressive and inborn autism, respectively.[41] In the accidental group, Down describes autistic symptoms in children who appear perfectly normal—the Virginia S. phenomenon—while lacking speech and displaying odd behaviors.

"They are bright in their expression, often active in their movements, agile to a degree, mobile in their temperament, fearless as to danger, persevering in mischief, petulant to have their own way. Their language is one of gesture only, living in a world of their own they are regardless of the ordinary circumstances around them." Down provides this one-sentence glimpse of a child who might have autism: "How the self-contained and self-absorbed little one cares not to be entertained other than in his own dreamland, and by automatic movements of his fingers or rhythmical movements of his body."

Because we don't know the developmental history of these children, the age of onset of their condition, or a more detailed set of behavior patterns, these could be true autism cases—among the few that caused us to pick the term "effectively zero" for the autism rate before 1930—or just the scattered presence of autistic traits (about which more in chapter 3). Some of these children, we argued in our book *The Age of Autism*, might have had a genetic disorder called Fragile X based on Down's description of their head shape. Interestingly, both Fragile X and Down are recognized today as risk factors for autism, so these children may have been especially susceptible to any number of environmental factors, not least of them London's famously dirty, coal-saturated air. (Recent studies have linked proximity to coal-fired plants to a doubled risk for autism.)

Down's cluster of possible autistic cases may have heralded the rise of the Age of Autism in the most vulnerable children in the most toxic-laden environments.

Potential cases, yes. Gulliver? Hardly.

◆ ◆ ◆

The earliest mentally retarded population on our list is Samuel Gridley Howe's. This is an especially interesting population because Donvan and Zucker trumpet Howe's report as a great discovery; they've been able to find evidence of autism in plain sight, they believe. Separate and apart from their book, *A Different Key,* they wrote about this discovery at some length in *Smithsonian* magazine, "The Early History of Autism."[42]

"Howe's 'Report Made to the Legislature of Massachusetts upon Idiocy,'" they write, "which he presented in February of 1848, includes signals of classic autistic behavior so breathtakingly recognizable to anyone familiar with the condition's manifestations that they cannot be ignored."

After hyping this glimpse of autism in nineteenth century America, they go on to stipulate how flimsy this evidence really is. "To be sure, Howe's cases do not prove there was a lot of autism in his day, or even any. But the concept of autism helps explain some of the cases that puzzled him."[43] Many careful authors qualify their assertions; few immediately trash the value of their "breathtaking" observation and suggest they "do not prove" a single solitary thing.

And did these cases really puzzle Howe, or are Donvan and Zucker making things up out of whole cloth? True to their pattern, the *Smithsonian* article invents a magical world of mystery and emotion. In typically fanciful prose, they describe the men from Boston arriving to examine one of their early autism candidates. "Billy was 59 years old that spring or summer of 1846, when a well-dressed man from Boston rode into his Massachusetts village on horseback, and began measuring and testing him in all sorts of ways. The visitor, as we imagine the scene, placed phrenologist's calipers on his skull, ran a tape measure around his chest and asked many questions relating to Billy's odder behaviors."

Donvan and Zucker imagine many things in their writing. But if one retraces their steps, it's easy to read the same document they read and upon close inspection conclude their "evidence" is far less compelling than their imagination.

Howe's actual report includes descriptions of 574 idiots, each one of which is examined and cataloged in a forty-page table at the end of the document. Four hundred twenty of these were truly idiots; 154 were regressive and showed a loss of skills. Howe also included most of these idiots in a systematic survey of mental retardation prevalence rates, one that spanned dozens of towns in Massachusetts. The geographic coverage of the prevalence survey wasn't entirely parallel with the individual case analyses of the 574, but 361 of these cases were in the towns surveyed.

The total population of the towns in the survey was 195,947; with 361 "idiots" this is a prevalence rate of 1 in 543, or less than 0.2 percent. This is already too small for Gulliver, but within his population of 574, barely 1 percent of those are even potentially autistic based on Donvan and Zucker's criteria.

Jonathan Rose, William R. Kenan Professor of History at Drew University whose calculations about Donald T.'s hometown we cited in the introduction, took on Donvan and Zucker's interpretation of the Howe data in a bracing article titled "Yes, There Is an Autism Epidemic"[44] on HistoryNewsNetwork.org.

"For most of the 574 'idiots' Howe surveyed, he doesn't offer enough information to make a conclusive diagnosis," Rose writes. "The data he does provide is occasionally consistent with autism, but also with other neurological disorders."[45]

We took a look at cases in Howe's sample that might be consistent with autism. There were six of them, and they were described with only the sketchiest of information. Howe devotes only page and a half to these cases. The most prominent of these is the aforementioned Billy, case number 27. From Howe: "This young man's sense of melody seems active and acute. He knows and can sing correctly more than 200 tunes. He will instantly detect a false note in any of them; yet he is an idiot in every other respect. If he is told to go and milk the cows, he stands and repeats over the words, 'Billy go and milk the cows,' for hours together or until someone tells him something else, which he will repeat over in the same way. But put a pail in his hand and make the sign for milking, and give him a push, and he will go and fill the pail."[46]

That's it. That's their best shot at describing a case of autism in Howe's study. Is it possible that Billy is autistic? Maybe. But there's nothing else in the description that provides a differential diagnosis between Billy's "idiocy" and many other potential diagnoses. Howe goes on to describe a number of other cases, most of which are described by savant skills. Case Number 360: "Tell him your age and ask him how many seconds it is and he will tell you in a very few minutes. In all other respects he is an idiot."[47]

"There are cases No. 175 and 192, idiots beyond all question, but who can count not only to 20 but to 20,000 and perform many simple arithmetical operations with a great deal more facility than ordinary persons."

Case Number 277: "A girl who can 'learn and know letters but can understand nothing of the subject to which they relate.'" Is this even a savant skill? Case Number 25 had a similarly limited capacity: "This young man knows the name and sound of every letter, he can put the letters into words, the words into sentences and read off a page with correctness; but he would read over that page a thousand times without getting the slightest idea of the meaning."

These six are possibly—but not persuasively—examples of the "idiot savant" phenomenon. This is a group that may have some overlap with autism but is generally accepted as not the same. What's more, even if all were autistic, these six cases constitute but 0.003 percent of the surveyed population—one in thirty-three thousand. This is the thin reed that Donvan and Zucker cling to as evidence of autism's historic presence, their best shot at finding Gulliver, and it collapses upon close inspection.

Jonathan Rose forcefully drives home the failure.

Thus the overwhelming preponderance of historical evidence indicates that the autism epidemic is all too real. Future historians will inevitably ask why so many public health officials and journalists refused to see the obvious and failed to pose some elementary questions about autism. Very likely there were some rare cases before the twentieth century, but in recent years the prevalence has skyrocketed. No doubt some individuals have a genetic predisposition to autism, but only environmental factors could have triggered such a sharp increase. Therefore, a prime goal of national health policy must be to identify those factors, eliminate them as far as possible, and roll back the epidemic. The well-being of future generations depends on that.[48]

Elsewhere, Donvan and Zucker go on to talk about wild children and holy fools as if these strange, random, celebrated cases somehow point to a significant substrate of fully autistic individuals. It's as if the presence of the bearded lady at the circus suggests the world is full of bearded ladies.

No, there's a reason people pay to see her. She's a rarity.

Insane Populations

If Gulliver can't be found in the intellectually disabled population, the next logical place to look for autism, as we've seen previously, is in populations of insane people. We've already described the rarity of childhood schizophrenia, so this quest is likely to be a fool's errand, but it is worth a quick review of some of the broader treatments of insane populations.

Perhaps the first of these is John Haslam, chief apothecary of the Bethlem Asylum, who wrote the first widely accepted description of madness in his 1809 monograph, *Observations on Madness and Melancholy.*[49] Across the channel in 1845, an early French psychiatrist named Jean-Étienne Esquirol wrote a book titled *Mental Maladies—a Treatise on Insanity,*[50] a comprehensive treatment of insanity in early nineteenth century France. Finally, Henry Maudsley, one of the more prominent experts, who now has a London psychiatric hospital named after him, wrote *The Physiology and Pathology of the Mind*[51] in 1867.

◆ ◆ ◆

The nineteenth century brought a flood of data, though not of cases, most notably in the descriptions of the "insane." William Haslam of

Bethlem Asylum in England (the famous "Bedlam") reported on a handful of cases among children. Two might have been autistic, but the etiology is at least as interesting as the evidence for autism.

"In the month of March 1799 a female child three and a quarter years old was brought in," Haslam wrote. "At 2 1/2 she was inoculated for smallpox. Severe convulsions ushered in the disease, and a delirium continued during its course.

"From the termination of the small-pox to the above date (nine months), the child continued in an insane state." Previously able to "articulate many words," she lost language, became violent, and would "rake out the fire with her fingers" despite getting burned. She would "bite, or express her anger by kicking or striking," and tried to run away.[52]

A second case, "a boy nearly 7 years of age was admitted into the hospital June 8, 1799. When a year-old he suffered much with the measles and afterward had a mild kind of inoculated smallpox." He became uncontrollable. Seen again at 15, he could whistle melodies but not answer questions, and had a fixation on toy soldiers.[53]

Perhaps we see why the Epidemic Denial authors glossed over these cases, as they point not just to symptoms but to environmental triggers. Genes that support a steady-state argument for autism's prevalence are the linchpin of the Epidemic Denial argument; environmental factors that could increase suddenly are anathema because they are consistent with a real rise in cases.

Jean-Étienne Esquirol, a pioneer in diagnosis and treatment of insanity in France, who in his 1845 book collected voluminous accounts of individual overall data over forty years, saw a wide range of insane patients but made the surprising claim that none of them were infants: "Infancy is secure from insanity, unless at birth, the child suffers from some vice of confirmation or convulsions, which occasion[s] imbecility or infancy."[54]

Esquirol goes on to cite Joseph Franck on a case from 1802 in London of "a child who had been a maniac from the age of two years," but Franck also commented on the rarity of such early cases. "He says, it is dementia only, that is not sometimes observed among the young, and only mania and melancholy, that do not appear in advanced life."[55] Unwound, that sentence says that young children never get dementia.

When they started to, around 1900, people like Weygandt and Heller noticed and scrambled to report it.

The Gulliver problem again: if infants are secure from dementia, and autism would surely have been considered a kind of dementia, what disorder do the Deniers think autism was hidden behind? As Leo Kanner himself later pointed out, in "the first 45 volumes of the *American Journal of Insanity* (1844–1889) there was not a single article pertaining to children."[56] Another doctor, Shobal V. Clevenger, compiled a review of the literature on mental illness in childhood from around the world in 1883 and found just fifty-five references.[57] And Edward Charles Spitza, in his "Treatment of Insanity" in the same year, declared infantile psychoses to be "rare and caused by heredity, fright, sudden changes of temperature or masturbation."[58] (If masturbation caused mental illnesses, they wouldn't be rare!)

Henry Maudsley wrote a chapter on "Insanity in Early Life" in his 1867 book on the pathology of the mind, and cited a thirdhand account of a child who was "raving mad as soon as it was born." The mother, however, "laughed and did the strangest things," suggesting a possible organic problem. In general, the ages of cases he describes in detail are the same range we have seen in other surveys.[59]

Maudsley lists as his chapter headings the kinds of madness to which children are vulnerable: Monomania or partial ideational insanity, Choric Delirium, Cateleptoid Insanity, Epileptic Insanity, Mania, Melancholia, Affective or Moral Insanity, Instinctive Insanity. As with Ireland's list, many suggest organic causes or injuries. A girl, age eight, became a "mischievous little machine, throwing everything down as soon as she got her hands on it"—but only after epilepsy that "produced an arrest of mental development." A boy, age ten, suffered a fall followed by headaches that led into convulsions and fits of involuntary laughter. Today we would probably treat this as a closed-head injury rather than any kind of mental problem.[60]

In summary, observers of insane populations—Haslam, Esquirol, and Maudsley—either report on the rarity of insanity in children or attribute a great deal of it to injury or disease. The timing of onset of these cases is random and scattered and includes a wide range of causal triggers including epilepsy, whooping cough, vaccination, or traumatic brain injury. In all, the evidence backs Esquirol's emphatic claim that "infancy is secure from insanity." No Gulliver here.

General Doctor's Patient Population

Finally, let's back up even further, to England in the 1600s, when a belief in "miasma" as the cause of disease and astrology and alchemy as treatment modalities still ruled the day; the idea of drinking mercuric chloride—a nasty concoction—had not yet happened. Around 1600, an astrologist-doctor named Richard Napier began treating adults and children at his office in Buckinghamshire, near London. Napier was organized and methodical—and that proved to be a gift to future medical historians. As Michael Macdonald writes in *Mystical Bedlam: Madness, Anxiety, and Healing in Seventeenth Century England*, "Like the buried remains of ancient nomads, the sources for the study of insanity are scattered and hidden in unlikely places."[61] Napier's practice was one.

From a start of merely treating neighbors, he ended up as a full-time practitioner and saw perhaps sixty thousand patients in thirty-seven years, taking careful notes on the symptoms the patients displayed. From this large sample of records, Macdonald extracted and analyzed the records of 2,483 mentally disturbed patients Napier saw over the course of a number of years; only 0.7 percent were children under ten. Today, they'd be well into double digits. In fact, out of all his young patients, half should have had a disability by today's insane levels. "The most striking feature of the distribution of ages among Napier's patients, both the physically ill and the mentally distressed, is the rarity of children among them," writes McDonald. "Disturbed children were strikingly rare among his clients."

Two centuries later, another location in London provided one of the "scattered and hidden" glimpses into children's mental health. At Great Ormond Street Hospital for Children, Dr. William Howship Dickinson, mostly known for his work in adult kidney problems, developed an interest in how ill health affected children's brains. A "meticulously careful observer," according to the Royal College of Physicians—shades of Napier—he left three volumes of handwritten case notes from 1861 to 1869 now in the hospital's Museum and Archives, providing vivid descriptions of 398 children with health issues that affected neurological functioning.

This group was examined by researchers Mitzi Waltz and Paul Shattock and written up in 2004 as "Autistic Disorder in Nineteenth Century London—Three Case Reports"[62] in *Autism: The International Journal of Research and Practice.* In all, the researchers found twenty-four cases in which "children presented with symptoms characteristic of autistic disorder," but when age of onset and lack of clear symptomatology were considered, Waltz and Shattock settled on two boys and one girl (who also had epilepsy) as meeting the criteria for a modern-day autism diagnosis.

"The existence of three relatively clear-cut cases of autism and numerous descriptions within a set of nineteenth-century medical notes will not surprise veteran researchers, many of whom mentioned pre-1943 cases that are consistent with autism."

Well, yes, it's not surprising to find three possible cases in a large children's hospital in the second half of the nineteenth century. This could again point to early effects of the industrial and medical industries—we've mentioned London's coal-fueled atmosphere, and the authors, note that mercury was used as a popular patent medicine for teething babies around that time. Many of the children also had bowel problems—frequently seen in today's autistic children—and were often treated with calomel, a mercury compound.

Such scattered cases arising in the nineteenth century before the first clear clusters begin in the 1930s point to the absence of evidence of anything like today's catastrophic autism rate. To borrow Tredgold's phrase about early hints of mental illness in children, they were "shadows of the coming event."

CHAPTER 3

Evidence of Absence:
The Empty Quadrant

"In some circumstances it can be safely assumed that if a certain event had occurred, evidence of it could be discovered by qualified investigators. In such circumstances it is perfectly reasonable to take the absence of proof of its occurrence as positive proof of its non-occurrence."
—*Copi, Introduction to Logic (1953)*[63]

I t is unusual to encounter a topic so important about which so much expert opinion is so dead, and as demonstrably and dangerously wrong as Autism Epidemic Denial. Part of our personal challenge as an autism parent and a health journalist becomes taking the "idea" seriously enough to debunk it thoroughly, not just wait for history to stomp all over nonsense as it is eventually wont to do.

Alas, we can't wait. Epidemic Denial does its damage daily. When Autism Speaks recently dropped its emphasis on looking for a "cure" for autism, Steve Silberman of *NeuroTribes* was ready with his Epidemic Denial shtick to help out. *New York* magazine, the equivalent of the cool-kids table for savvy Manhattanites, took note of it this way:

"'This is a big deal—or, rather, it could be,' said Steve Silberman," because talking about a cure distracted from the scientific evidence that has called into question that notion of autism as an 'epidemic.' As he details in his best-selling book, what seemed like a sudden and inexplicable increase in children with autism can be explained by the arrival of three important changes that all happened around the same time: 'radically broadened diagnostic criteria, more widely available screening tests, and greater community awareness of the condition.'"[64]

We called that a flavor of denial—"science" has spoken—in the introduction. Here we see how pernicious it is: Because autism hasn't really increased, the argument goes, we don't need to look for a cause or cure for a human variation that is proving surprisingly adaptive in today's wired world. We just need to get used to it. No wonder *Wired*, the *New York* of Silicon Valley, published Silberman's goofy "The Geek Syndrome"[65] in 2001. It posited that "assortative mating" of previously unmarriageable nerds flocking to Silicon Valley led to more extreme forms of nerdiness in their offspring—a.k.a. autism. What we really need, by this reckoning, is to let Asperger's kids fix our computers and musical savants make us weep.

◆ ◆ ◆

So Epidemic Denial and its awful implications depend on the intellectually flaccid assumption of autism as a world historical constant, not a worldwide environmental catastrophe. That explains our humble efforts in the midst of all this celebration to turn up anything close to the billion and a half people who should have lived on Earth before 1930 if the autism prevalence rate has stayed steady through human history. We found surpassingly few in populations where there should have been millions. We invoked Gulliver as our autism mascot because among the very rare childhood diseases of the early twentieth century, Gulliver—autism—should have dwarfed all else. You wouldn't need a new diagnostic category or greater awareness to hear his lumbering feet nearby; you couldn't miss them.

But there is one more pathway into the past that has a chance of leading to individual cases of autism—though hardly a hidden horde of Gulliverian proportions. We want to take a methodical look at medical case studies of children with any kind of intellectual or developmental problem before 1930. We want to see if autism as defined today could be present in any of them.

First, we'll offer a sometimes neglected detail—a careful description of how a case of autism is defined, building on Leo Kanner's 1943 paper but relying on the written criteria established in the mid-1970s and prevailing until 2013's DSM-V (the Diagnostic and Statistical Manual of Mental Disorders, Version V). That version departed in some respects from the standard and long-standing definitions, but it is so recent it has nothing to do with any increase. Then we'll take a deep dive—far deeper than the Deniers have ever immersed themselves—in the historical literature of children's mental disorders and see how many autism cases we can surface.

We hope that unless you have a personal or professional interest in denying the truth, you will agree that whatever turns up, on top of last chapter's broader search of populations and diagnoses and chapter 1's look at very rare early childhood disorders that had been fully characterized decades before, constitutes a fair and full attempt to locate autism before 1930. Let the cases surface where they may and the false assumptions, whatever they turn out to be, fall away.

◆ ◆ ◆

Building a Fence Around Autism

Retrospective diagnosis is difficult, and we are not diagnosticians, so we don't claim to be doing any diagnoses other than whether a case is plausibly autistic, with the benefit of the doubt going to the notion that it is. As you've seen, we believe the most useful criterion is age of onset, and we'll rely on that as our baseline requirement.

The other criterion is the belief that turning to qualified investigators—as in the epigraph for this chapter—is the best bet. Your uncle may think Isaac Newton or his father's car repairman was autistic, but we don't care what your uncle thinks and, frankly, neither should you. Instead, we'll look in the published medical literature for case reports—the raw material there is voluminous. In chapter 1, we saw that two qualified investigators were fully able to detect and diagnose the rare disorder named for them—Heller-Weygandt, a.k.a. *dementia infantilis*—and that other investigators took the rare measure of childhood schizophrenia. Meanwhile, large populations like the mentally disabled and those living in asylums were carefully surveyed and described by a whole range of investigators. Even among those we would today call family practitioners or GPs, some had careful records going back centuries that contained little to no hint of autism.

Qualified investigators, in short, came up with nothing, which is strong evidence, according to the *Introduction to Logic,* that there *was* nothing—which is our thesis: before 1930, the rate of autism in the world was effectively zero. This sounds extreme. The qualification *effectively* is important. That doesn't mean absolutely zero. Today, we are looking at 1.5 percent of children with autism; within a short period after Kanner discovered it, the rate was around 0.01 percent—one in ten thousand. One in ten million, which may very well have been the rate for millennia before that, is 0.00001 percent (that rate would have given us a dozen cases in the United States and three dozen in Europe). How many zeros standing in formation do we have to march past like the queen reviewing the Royal Guard before we arrive at *effectively* zero? This many, we'd say.

So by all means, hold us to the marker we've put down but also understand the significance if we're right: The paucity of cases before 1930, followed by the first clusters, followed by a slow rise, followed by today's catastrophic numbers, means autism is a new, disabling, environmentally triggered disorder—an *epidemic* disorder. When Leo Kanner reported on the first cases, the eldest was born in 1931. He believed their disorder was new, and he never reported on an earlier birth year for an autistic child despite several decades as a world "clearing house" for cases. (Hans Asperger will occupy the next chapter.)

There's a reason this is controversial, as the *New York* article illustrates. It matters because it means something changed in the environment to trigger those first few cases and the subsequent deluge. *What* changed is not our topic here; *that* it changed is. The simple fact points to a terrifying environmental epidemic, utterly opposite to the warm and fuzzy orthodoxy peddled by *In a Different Key* and *NeuroTribes* and their ilk.

As we look for cases of autism before 1930, then, it is critical to spell out precisely what an autism diagnosis involves. As we've seen, the language of psychiatry is clogged with nomenclature and distinctions without a difference to normal observers (hebephrenic, parergastic?) We've tried to come up with a simple but accurate way to understand it. Any diagnosis is differential—it sets the disorder or disability apart from normal functioning and also from previously described disorders that were the most similar. Autism can seem confounding both because it is a "spectrum" disorder in which some people are severely affected and others function reasonably well, and because the criteria for the disorder—the length of the spectrum, you might say—has changed over the years in ways that some claim explain the greatly increasing numbers. This is false, as we'll show.

So think of a diagnosis as a confined space inhabited by people who are alike in a set of crucial ways, bounded by lines that rule all others out. People with autism and only people with autism go inside our enclosure; others of whatever description can roam anywhere else they please. (And note: we are not "corralling" autistic individuals, just using the sharpest visual imagery we can think of to avoid the jargon that tends to favor Denier mush.)

Let's start at the beginning and stake the first autism fence posts around Leo Kanner's 1943 paper, in which he grouped the eleven children he observed as "markedly and uniquely different from anything reported so far." In what way, we need to ask, were they markedly and uniquely different? Kanner did not systematize his observations, but he did describe in remarkable and enduring detail their most distinctive and striking features. "The combination of extreme autism [the trait of aloneness, self-involvement], obsessiveness, stereotypy and echolalia bring the total picture into relationship with some of the basic schizophrenia phenomena," he wrote in 1943. "Some of the children have indeed been diagnosed as this type at one time or another. But in spite of the remarkable similarities, the condition differs in many respects from all other known instances of childhood schizophrenia."[66]

So Kanner calls out social aloofness, language oddities, and obsessiveness as the essence of the behavioral syndrome. Kanner was working in the community of child psychiatrists; other conditions of children, most notably *dementia infantilis* (the more obscure label *dementia praecocissimia* was generally considered the same disorder) and childhood schizophrenia were well-known. The final feature that distinguished it from these others is the age of onset. In his original paper, he gives it primacy:

"First of all, even in cases with the earliest recorded onset of schizophrenia, including those of De Sanctis's *dementia praecocissemia* and of Heller's *dementia infantilis,* the first observable manifestations were preceded by at least two years of essentially average development; the histories specifically emphasize a more or less gradual *change* in the patient's behavior. The children of our group have all shown their extreme aloneness from the very beginning of life, not responding to anything that comes to them from the outside world." Given that characteristic and extreme *aloneness,* Kanner borrows Bleuler's *autismus* from 1911 and elevates it from a trait to the name of the disorder. (In this paper he talks about "autistic disturbances"; in a 1944 paper he settles on the term "early infantile autism," again pointing to the extremely young age of onset of those who fit within the diagnosis.[67])

So let's build up the boundaries from Kanner's original descriptions.

- Extreme aloneness or autism, the characteristic deficit of the disorder.
- Evident "from the very beginning of life" (later, the first two years of infancy).
- "Anxiously obsessive desire for the maintenance of sameness that nobody but the child himself may disrupt on occasion." These are traits of obsessiveness and stereotypy, a narrow range of interests, whether train schedules, Disney characters, or the weather. This is the one most commonly shared with Asperger's and is often not disabling by itself.
- Lack of functional language: some of Kanner's children never spoke at all; none used language the way the rest of us do.

"From the start language—which the children did not use for the purposes of communication—was deflected in a considerable measure to a self-sufficient semantically and conversationally valueless or grossly distorted memory exercise," he wrote. These abnormalities extended to pronoun reversal ("You fall down," Case 1 said to his mother when *he* fell down) and echolalia (repeating what was said, some of it from advertisements or jingles, without understanding what was meant and often with considerable delay).

So Kanner stakes four fence posts that create the boundaries of the autism enclosure: age of onset, lack of functional language, extreme aloneness, and preservation of sameness. In 1956, he and his colleague Leon Eisenberg tried to boil it all down to "extreme self-isolation and the obsessive insistence on the preservation of sameness."[68] They mentioned for the first time that regressive cases—up to eighteen to twenty months—had started to present themselves. But the basic enclosure prevailed and made it hard from the very beginning to miss the cases that belonged within it. You were autistic, or you were not.

By 1978, as cases slowly became more noticeable in the practices of child psychiatry, British psychiatrist Michael Rutter codified the condition.[69] He moved the age of onset to thirty months or younger—two and a half years. This had the benefit of capturing regressive cases that had continued to increase, as well as setting autism apart from *dementia infantilis,* which usually was seen at ages four or five but sometimes described as occurring, imprecisely, "during the third year of life." Ages six, seven, or eight might be the rare cases of childhood schizophrenia (so rare that many doubted its existence); ten or above, standard onset schizophrenia.

Rutter states the following:

In summary the definition of childhood autism in terms of four essential criteria in relation to the child's behavior before age five [when a diagnosis can safely be made based on behavior apparent at 30 months] still seems to be the best procedure. The four criteria are (1) an onset before the age of 30 months; (2) impaired social development which has a number of special characteristics and which is out of keeping with the child's intellectual level; (3) delayed and deviant language development which also has certain defined features and which is out of keeping with the child's intellectual level, and (4) 'insistence on sameness' as shown by stereotyped play patterns, abnormal preoccupations, or resistance to change. The syndrome as defined in this way has been shown to be valid and meaningful in that it differs markedly from other clinical syndromes in a host of respects. It is strongly recommended that, in order to insure comparability, all investigators define their samples in this way.[70]

(Note that Rutter in 1955 uses the same word as Kanner in 1943—"markedly"—to show how strongly autism differed from other disorders in "a host of respects.")

As he set the thirty-month limit for autism, Rutter described studies from the 1960s and 1970s on "the age distribution for onset of psychoses in childhood." Interestingly, this shows a sharp change in distribution from the early twentieth century we examined in chapter 1. It is more strong evidence that autism was a new arrival.

"There is one large peak for children whose disorders begin before three years of age and a second large peak for those whose psychoses are evident in early adolescence or shortly before that. Psychosis beginning in middle childhood is much rarer." The latter is a clear reference to Heller's *dementia infantilis*. This passage is evidence that the dominant diagnoses of the early twentieth century—Heller's disease and childhood schizophrenia—have vanished from the field of view almost entirely. They were always rare, and now the field is dominated

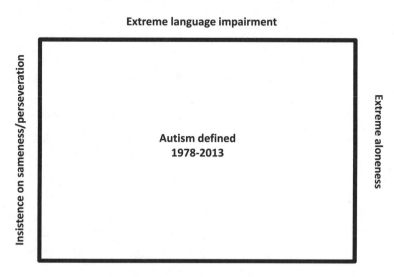

by regular adolescent-onset schizophrenia, which had long been recognized, and by autism, which was new.[71]

We'll examine how Rutter's official boundaries changed, but for now it is important to recognize that first Kanner, and then Rutter, differentiated autism from childhood schizophrenia and Heller's. Kanner, in setting apart autism as "markedly and uniquely different" in 1943, explicitly differentiated the two conditions. He distinguishes his case series from them with the age of onset, among other defining features. Having written the book in 1935 on childhood mental disorders, one could hardly ask for a more authoritative source to make these distinctions. Rutter also differentiated autism from other "disintegrative disorders" (citing Heller), but by 1978, the term *dementia infantilis* didn't even merit a mention in Rutter's account.

Donvan and Zucker and Silberman try to push back against this powerful evidence in the only way possible. They assert Kanner didn't believe autism was new, ignoring his multiple published statements of exactly that belief and quoting a 1969 speech to autism parents in which he said, "I did not discover autism. It was there before." That was the same speech in which he falsely stated he had never blamed parents for inducing the condition, laid the responsibility on Bruno Bettelheim (who richly deserved the lion's share), and told the assembled crowd, "I hereby acquit you people," whereas the proper stance might have been to ask "you people" for forgiveness.[72]

Whatever Kanner may have meant in this after-dinner talk (if we were Donvan and Zucker, we might imagine him in an expansive mood with drink in hand and his reliable cigar, saying things he'd never write in a medical journal), it seemed designed to ingratiate himself with autism parents. Saying autism "was there before" could have been another way of lifting the blame off that generation of parents, among whom were a high number of college-educated mothers joining the workforce for the first time whom he had viewed with suspicion. Or he may simply have acknowledged what we do, that scattered cases existed before 1930—he had already mentioned Weygandt's cases as early evidence of autism—though as we've seen, that's an imprecise comparison. Yet a decade after his dinner comment he repeated his statement that autism was "unknown to me or anyone else theretofore."

Zucker and Donvan, surviving as they must on such thin gruel in their attempt to treat autism as ancient, try to make a meal of autism being "there before." Kanner, among thousands of other observers over hundreds of years, just saw it clearly for the first time, that's all. They wrote, "It was Kanner who identified the two defining traits common to all of them: the extreme preference for aloneness and the extreme need for sameness. It was this pairing of extremes, he decided, that formed the heart of the syndrome he was talking about, whose presence had previously been masked by the differences among the children.

"It was there before."[73]

Apparently, Kanner could write five hundred pages in 1935 on every conceivable disorder but miss this most common one, the one with the earliest onset and the most striking symptoms. These amazing behaviors, which struck him emphatically when he saw the first children in 1930s, had been masked by—well, by what exactly? Donvan and Zucker point to the fact that Kanner himself says some of these children would have had an initial diagnosis of childhood schizophrenia, or the comment about Weygandt, but they ignore the later onset and rarity of both.

We'll show how the boundaries of the diagnosis of autism did change, along with the words used to describe it, but how little that mattered. Once cases began after 1930, autism remained autism. Identifiable. Impossible to ignore. Increasing. Intriguing to any specialist in the field of child psychiatry. After 1930, qualified investigators were there to document autism's reality and its rise. Before 1930, qualified investigators found barely a trace.

Case Control

What Epidemic Deniers so desperately need are cases that fit within our "autism corral"—the boundaries constructed by Kanner. It's an extraordinary claim that autism was always there, long before Kanner and Asperger labeled it. So it's not enough just to say, "here are traits." It's important to describe an individual who meets the boundary fence criteria: plausible presence of all three impairments and an age of onset before thirty to thirty-six months. Whereas the early observers of schizophrenia and idiocy tended to devote most of their writing to broad strokes and theory, there is also a substantial literature that goes deep on cases.

We had run into this literature before, as we explored evidence of cases before 1930 for our first book. But with the new claims from the Deniers, we decided to go deeper. We realized that Kanner wasn't the first person to describe case series. Heller and Weygandt did it, as we've seen, and many others did the same thing. In fact, we ran into case descriptions so frequently in the literature that we decided one way to approach the argument was to collect a sample of these case descriptions of mentally ill children in a more organized way. We knew from experience that case descriptions could run from a few sentences to a few paragraphs to several pages at a time. What was most important was the breadth of the information on each child. We even ran into one case description that went on for six whole articles.

So we went on a comprehensive search for articles where there was a plausible individual description of a case of autism before Kanner and Asperger. The questions we needed to answer for the articles that met our search criteria were simple:

- Was the child born before or after 1930? To specify the time of birth, we collected birth years when available and estimated them when reasonable, using publication year, information on the age of the children, and giving a little time for the publication process.
- Was the child described with relevant autistic traits? We didn't set the bar especially high here; if we could find plausible evidence of autistic traits, we included the case. We excluded case reports that included prominent mention of some kind of meningitis, encephalitis, or brain injury.
- Was the age of onset before or after thirty months of age? We decided to use thirty months because while Heller's disease has its onset in the "third or fourth year of life," we found no mentions of Heller's onset earlier than two and a half years of age. And we have found very few autism cases before or since when the actual onset is not evident well before thirty months—most frequently, regressive cases show themselves starkly by a year and a half to two years of age. We also found and included a number

of cases with later onset than *dementia infantilis*; many of these had been placed under the childhood schizophrenia label.

We then went searching for articles with in-depth descriptions of individual cases among which there might have been a plausible case of autism. Within this collection of plausible cases, our key screening criterion for an autism case was simple—the age of onset was before thirty months of age. In building out our plausible case sample, we looked for relevant citations in several places:

1. Silberman's sources. He cited a number of articles in *NeuroTribes* as evidence for early autism cases; most of these were derived from an academic review article by Shorter and Wachtel,[74] so we included sources from Shorter and Wachtel as well.

2. Donvan and Zucker's sources. This wasn't hard, since *In a Different Key* only mentioned the Howe cases in Massachusetts in the 1800s, a handful with savant traits and no detailed description. They also mentioned Archie Casto, a possible case born before 1930, but there is no evidence beyond his deceased mother's recollection.

3. Leo Kanner's articles and textbooks. As we've mentioned, before Kanner saw Case 1, Donald Triplett, in 1938, he had written the first English language textbook on child psychiatry in 1935.[75] We looked for citations in his section on "major psychoses" in that edition. We also looked at his revised section on Heller's in the 1967 edition.[76] In terms of his articles, we looked for citations from his 1943 paper as well as extracting individual case descriptions from his later papers.

4. R. A. Q. Lay's 1938 review. In a helpful coincidence, his 1938 paper gave an exhaustive survey of the literature on "schizophrenia-like psychoses in young children." This would be a terrific place to find mentions of unlabeled autism. We cited this review in *The Age of Autism*, but this time, we dug into his citations. Lay also provided six detailed case descriptions of his own.

5. Our previous research. In writing *The Age of Autism*, we collected relevant case histories from a number of sources, including

Bernie Rimland's 1964 book *Infantile Autism.*[77] We reviewed all of those sources and revisited their case histories in greater depth.

6. Other prominent observers. As we conducted this review, we encountered other leading diagnosticians who had addressed the topic, including Lorna Wing and Arn van Krevelen; we reviewed their articles for additional evidence and potential cases.

It was a fascinating body of literature, evenly divided between English and German (mostly untranslated, our colleague Birgit Calhoun again proving invaluable with her translations from German) with a couple of Italian journals thrown in. Publication dates ranged from 1906 to 1972.

In total, we reviewed around forty studies; twenty-nine of these had enough case information to make a determination of autism, and from these twenty-nine publications we extracted a total of ninety-one cases born between 1890 and 1950. The vast majority described a regressive pattern of onset. Of these ninety-one cases, almost all with a year of birth before 1930 described the age of onset at between thirty months

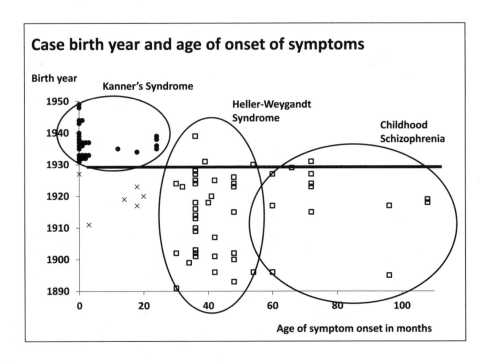

Case birth year and age of onset of symptoms

and ten years—putting them outside the range of an autism diagnosis. Most of these cases fit the Heller-Weygandt description. We did find a number of cases with an early age of onset (i.e., before thirty months); but with a few exceptions, these cases were born after 1930.

In order to visualize how these cases met or failed to meet the Epidemic Denier hypothesis, we plotted them on a chart, including the age of onset of their disorder on the horizontal (left-right) axis and year of birth on the vertical (up-down) axis. We included birth years between 1890 and 1950, since most of the case reports we uncovered were published in the twentieth century. In the first chart we included age of onset up to ten years of age (120 months at the far lower right).

At the top left, in the area that comprises the earliest age of onset and the most recent in terms of year of observation, you'll see the grouping of clear-cut autism cases plotted as round dots. Those include Kanner's original eleven autism cases, a number of new case descriptions from his 1972 paper,[78] as well as cases from other authors,[79] including Group 1 from the paper by Lauretta Bender in 1947.[80] Moving a little to the right—to the later age of onset on the left-right axis—are Heller-Weygandt syndrome cases that we have discussed in detail (Bender also described these in her paper, as Group 2). They were rare, and you may recall that Heller in 1930 had managed to collect only twenty-eight cases since 1906, when he observed the first one.

Moving further to the right—to even later in terms of age of onset— are the even rarer cases of childhood schizophrenia, those with onset before puberty (Bender's Group 3). We've plotted the later age of onset cases as small squares.

The lower left, below 1930 and under thirty months of age, is where Epidemic Deniers claim the hidden horde existed—this is where Gulliver should be crouched in the shadows in the form of children with autism symptoms, manifesting before thirty months of age. As you can see, this is hardly teeming with cases. In fact, we call it the Empty Quadrant. Even by the standards of rarity set by Heller-Weygandt syndrome and childhood schizophrenia, it is notably without observation of anything at all before 1930, when it suddenly kicks up and overtakes the other two disorders (our graph, which ends in 1950, tracks only the start of autism's rise, of course).

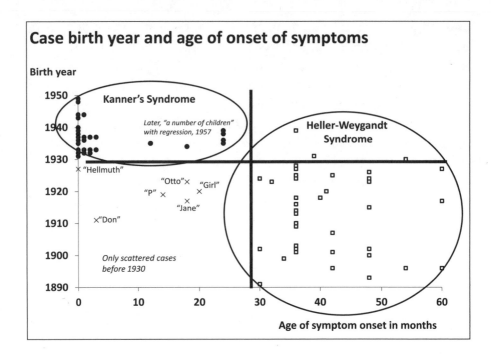

Case birth year and age of onset of symptoms

Birth year

Kanner's Syndrome

Later, "a number of children" with regression, 1957

Heller-Weygandt Syndrome

× "Hellmuth"

"Otto"× "Girl"
"P" × ×
× "Jane"

× "Don"

Only scattered cases before 1930

Age of symptom onset in months

The Empty Quadrant is so empty there is not even anything to *confuse* with autism. Remember Esquirol in 1845? "Infancy is secure from insanity" barring some external mishap. That held through 1930, when it gave way in a rush.

As you can also see, the Empty Quarter is effectively but not utterly empty. We've marked six plausibly autistic case studies with light blue Xs that met the Epidemic Deniers' hypothesis—born before 1930 with onset before thirty months. In order to visualize the nature of this group, we zoomed in and limited the oldest age on the chart to sixty months; this allows a more granular look at the lower-left Empty Quarter—we've named each of them when the case study we're referring to does so. The bottom line, quite literally: where all those supposed autism cases should be hiding, we see only scattered cases before 1930 that might fit the Deniers' bill.

Between 1890 and 1930, we find six possible cases with onset before thirty months; one of those, Hellmuth, is a case described in Asperger's 1944 paper and five are individual cases. Along the boundary that lies closest to the Empty Quadrant, there are relatively few cases as well, only nine with an onset starting at thirty months up to thirty-five months (these are the earliest onset cases of *dementia infantilis*); from thirty-six months to ten years of age we found forty-four—most of those typical Heller's with a few cases of childhood schizophrenia thrown in.

A few caveats. We have mentioned earlier a few scattered cases that were born before 1890. These included Waltz and Shattuck's three retrospective diagnoses (found in William Howship Dickinson's medical notes) and John Haslam's two children who became "insane" after vaccination (at Bethlem Asylum). Both were younger than thirty months, which plants them firmly in autism-onset territory. We don't display these on the graph but will include them in our final tally.

We also excluded from the chart six "Little Professors" similar to Asperger's reports in Russia by Sukhareva,[81] about which more will be discussed in upcoming chapters.

As for the other quadrants, the upper left clearly describes autism as we know it. And the quadrants on the right (both the zoomed out and zoomed in versions) included the rare but well-documented disorders *dementia infantilis* and childhood schizophrenia. Having immersed ourselves in the early twentieth century literature of childhood onset mental disorders, these two conditions stood out like giants; anyone who was anyone in the field knew and described these disorders fluently. Ultimately, however, the Gulliver of autism swallowed these smaller disorders altogether. Childhood schizophrenia, always so rare its existence was suspect, stood alongside autism for a while before it was jettisoned: what was once the *Journal of Autism and Childhood Schizophrenia* was renamed the *Journal of Autism and Developmental Disabilities* in 1979. And what was first called *dementia infantilis* was later called childhood disintegrative disorder and included in the Pervasive Developmental Disorders. In 2013, however, Childhood Disintegrative Disorder vanished into oblivion in the vastness of Autistic Spectrum Disorder in the *Diagnostic and Statistical Manual Version V*. Today, only Gulliver is left, overshadowing everything, impossible to miss.

Getting Granular

Now let's home in on the handful of cases scattered around the Empty Quadrant that might conceivably be autistic. We have found just a half dozen of these, but in numerous respects their unique case histories suggest something different than autism as Kanner described it, whether is from be an infection, a toxic exposure, or it is a collection of symptoms that doesn't match the level of disability we see in a typical case. Let's review each these cases in depth.

Don

In 1920, a Philadelphia psychiatrist, Lightner Witmer, wrote at some length of "A Curable Case Of Arrested Development Due To A Fear Of Psychosis the Result Of A Shock In A Three-Year-Old Infant."[82] We first came upon Witmer's account in Bernie Rimland's 1964 book *Infantile Autism,* where Rimland wrote, "Witmer (1920) described a severely afflicted three-year-old boy who appeared in many ways to resemble the autistic cases of Kanner. At age seven, Witmer's case seemed destined to recover."[83] Witmer wrote about a boy named Don, born in 1917, who "had to be taught to crawl and to walk, and even then he could only toddle around uncertainly." Don "never uttered a word spontaneously." In Witmer's elaborate account, Don exhibited clear signs of autistic aloneness.

"I saw Donald for the first time when he was two years and seven months old [in 1919]," wrote Witmer. "His father carried him into the office, and deposited him, a soulless lump, upon the couch. He sat there with the stolidity of a Buddhist image, absorbed in the inspection of a card he held in his pudgy hands, as regardless of his father and mother as of the new objects around him."

His overall physical development was profoundly delayed, Witmer recounted. But there were other, organic possibilities.

"He had an illness after birth," Witmer wrote of Don, "which I now believe left his brain so devitalized that it permitted fear to gain the upper hand over desire."[84] But what was the "shock" at age three to which Witmer refers in his title? In a footnote Rimland may have overlooked, Witmer notes that while "the etiology is uncertain, something like hydrocephaly was suspected but rejected as the explanatory cause. It may have been nutrition, but I incline to believe it was only the shock of an attack of whooping cough."

Post-pertussis encephalitis is a well-known cause of brain damage, and may explain a number of early cases about which we have limited information. In 1942, Louis A. Lurie and Sol Levy, writing in the *Journal of the American Medical Association,* noted "personality changes and behavior disorders which may occur in children many years following an attack of whooping cough suffered early in infancy."[85] In a study of five hundred "problem children," 243 or 48.6 percent were found to have had whooping cough. Of those, fifty-eight were two years or younger at the time, and in a third of those "there appeared to be a definite relationship between the neurological sequelae of the whooping cough and the behavior disorders and personality changes shown by them in later life."

So in a case of someone born before 1930 showing mental disturbances, but lacking a detailed mental history, the possibility of brain damage from a disease cannot be ruled out. Similarly, C. L. Davidson and Jean Terry Thomas wrote in 1948 in *Archives of Disease in Childhood* that "encephalitis has now been recognized for many years as a rare but serious complication of vaccination and some hundreds of cases have been reported."[86] They called the incidence "extremely rare in the first year of life," though the case history they described was four months old. Mental illness in children was also extremely rare in the first year of life before 1930. How many cases of plausible autism—like the cases reported by Haslam—might involve encephalitis induced by illness or vaccination is unknowable but needs to be considered.

Was Don truly autistic, as Rimland suggested, or simply suffering from a brain injury incurred during an illness? We suspect the latter.

Jane

Kanner himself cited one pre-1930 child as autistic—a girl named Jane described in "Case Report Twenty-Eight Years After an Infantile Autistic Disorder" by George C. Darr and Frederic G. Worden.[87] Darr and Worden reported on a case first seen by their colleagues. "In 1921 a four-year-old girl was brought to the Henry Phipps Psychiatric Clinic of the Johns Hopkins Hospital. From the descriptions by Dr. Adolf Meyer and Dr. Esther Richards, who saw her, it is apparent that the child presented a syndrome now called early infantile autism."[88]

Kanner wrote a commentary on Darr and Worden's paper and posed a provocative issue. "The question has often been raised: What becomes of autistic children when they grow up?" To our knowledge, he never reported on an adult case born earlier than his own cases, but he used this opportunity to observe a supposed adult case to argue for the importance of his newfound diagnostic framework. Since "the syndrome of early infantile autism was not separated from the multitude of child psychoses until less than fifteen years ago . . . [it is no] wonder that psychiatrists of the caliber of Drs. Meyer and Richards felt that they were dealing with something unique, with something which they had not encountered before and for which they had no frame of diagnostic reference."

Adolf Meyer, as we mentioned earlier, was Kanner's mentor, and Esther Richards was a colleague (she spotted Virginia S., one of the original autism cases, in a home for feeble-minded children, and described her as "completely different from all the others").

But was Jane really autistic? While certain features of the case are consistent with autism—the child "does not look into people's eyes"; "nothing makes a great deal of difference"; she is "not much affected by stimuli"; "is afraid of certain objects (e.g., the stove)"—other aspects are not. As a teenager, she "had to be admitted to the disturbed ward of a mental hospital because of confused episodes, periods of excitement, threatening to jump out of the windows, feeling that she was being poisoned, that she was full of gas, and that there was no oxygen in her blood. . . . She explained at length in fairly friendly fashion that she had chemical poisons within her and that if she lit a match she would explode." Delusions, or any description of inner life, are simply not characteristic of children with autism. Kanner later said that as his own cases grew older, he never saw a single episode of delusions or hallucinations.

Upon close inspection, it's not at all clear that Jane was a typical case of autism. She played piano with some skill and learned fluent Spanish, suggesting less language impairment than one would usually expect in autism. She achieved a notable degree of independence and "was sent to live with a series of four companions . . . either traveling or living in city apartments with them. . . . She was able to take care of her own personal needs. She could come and go alone about the city. She continued taking piano and voice lessons, attended concerts frequently, enjoyed movies, dancing and entertaining with her companions in her apartment."

There is little doubt that Jane was a troubled young woman. Some of her delusional symptoms suggest schizophrenia more than autism. Or perhaps she wasn't delusional at all: maybe her claims of being poisoned meant she really was dealing with a toxic exposure of some kind. It's hard to draw definitive conclusions from the description.

Was Jane really autistic as Kanner asserted? Or was he eager to make the case for his new syndrome and force fit the label on a more complex case? We don't believe the answer is clear here either way.

Otto

Otto, as recounted by J. Lutz, was born March 3, 1923. Unlike the cases of Don and Jane, Otto's description is brief, just 150 words or so. According to Lutz, his symptoms began in the second year of life, including language peculiarities, grimacing, dissociation, and psychosis. He was able to start school at six but had what Lutz called "phonographism"—he reproduced everything he heard at school. "Contact was disturbed in the most severe sense—dissociated, ambivalent, negativistic. Disturbed motor function. Language actually intact."[89]

Lutz called it "an insidiously progressive early childhood form of psychosis." The onset was early, but was it autism? The grimacing recalls Heller-Weygandt syndrome. Otto may have met the criteria for an autism diagnosis today, but he was by no means a typical case.

"Girl"

Another brief description, this one slightly longer at just over five hundred words, came from Dr. Herbert Jancke in Bonn, Germany. In a 1929 article on Heller's syndrome entitled, "Two Cases of Dementia Infantilis,"[90] the first of Jancke's cases presented with an age of onset that was earlier than normal for *dementia infantilis*.

Like most cases of Heller's, the girl developed typically. "After a normal birth the patient developed very well, said a few words already at 9 months, played with the mother in a room at 1 year 6 months and got herself her own food. Today the parents are of the opinion that she was intellectually precocious."

Then she regressed. "At 1 year 8 months the parents noticed that her state was not quite normal. She started, without ever having been physically ill, to tilt the head to the side putting the finger on the temple and perform slow (athetoid) movements with hands and arms. She lost her ability to speak; the language became more and more inarticulate, the child more and more restless, it constantly ran around in the room and, from time to time uttered screams, started to grind her teeth, pushed her lower jaw forward, implement chewing movements, and utter sounds that were reminiscent of the Germanic 'eh.'"

The office visit described her symptoms. Some seem consistent with autism, such as stimming behavior, "never ending movements of any one body part at variable speeds some of which keep re-occurring such as the laying over of the thumb over the index finger." Others sound more like Heller's: "The facial musculature displays grimacing twitches, the child grinds the teeth, babbles, hums, and utters individual screams."

Was "Girl" an early case of autism or simply an unusually early onset case of *dementia infantilis?* One could make an argument either way.

Hellmuth

Hellmuth was one of the four cases from Asperger's landmark 1944 paper. He appears to have been born in the mid- to late 1920s, several years earlier than the other three, and was different from them in other key respects. Asperger described Hellmuth as "grotesquely fat" and reports a likely brain injury at birth. He "had severe asphyxia at birth and was resuscitated at length. Soon after his birth he had convulsions, which recurred twice within the next few days but have not since." He was delayed physically, starting to walk and talk only at the end of his second year. "However, he then learnt to speak relatively quickly, and even as a toddler he talked 'like a grown-up.' . . . On top of the massive body, over the big face with flabby cheeks, was a tiny skull. One could almost consider him microcephalic."

Hellmuth also had a complex range of medical problems, in addition to his obesity, which continued "despite a strict, medically supervised diet. He gained weight without having a big appetite . . . he had distinctly formed 'breasts and hips.'" He had two undescended testicles and "had been treated with hormone preparations."

Asperger himself put Hellmuth in a different category. "In Hellmuth's case, there were clear indications that his autism was due to brain injury at birth. . . . His medical history—asphyxia, fits, endocrine disorder, hyper-salivation, neurologically based apraxia—clearly pointed to an organic cause."[91]

So does Hellmuth really belong in the Empty Quadrant? Despite his status as the sole member of the original Asperger case series born before 1930, he appears to be an outlier in this group, which would make Asperger's true case series of "idiopathic autism" really a series of three.

P

As far as we know, P's case is the single most extensive early onset regressive description before 1930 available to medicine; it was considered so notable at the time it ran as a five-part series. We believe we have obtained the first English translation of the article series, which was authored in 1931 by Swiss psychiatrist N. Moritz Tramer, and titled "Tagebuch über ein geistekrankes Kind," or "Diary About a Mentally Ill Child."[92] It is based on P.'s mother's journal entries, which began well before he regressed and continued until he was not quite five. There was clearly an early and complicated onset, but also one with a possible environmental trigger, just as we've seen in several other possible early cases of autism. P was born in 1919, and according to Tramer, the "start of the illness falls . . . into the 2nd year of life." This would make P a candidate to occupy the Empty Quadrant.

At eleven months, P. had what Tramer described as a "reaction to a railroad trip." His development until then had been normal, and he liked the train rides he had experienced up to that point.

"On the first evening he couldn't sleep in the dark," his mother wrote. "He was too excited about the many new impressions. When he was among strangers for a while and then saw me suddenly, he stretched both arms more vehemently to me, pulled my sleeves down to him-self and burrowed his little head into my neck. Since we have gotten home again, these downright passionate eruptions of tenderness are not happening. Our relationship is quieter again. He stands firmly on his legs and expresses an immense joy when I let him 'walk' a little by lifting him up like a little doll and then put him down again. That one could move one's own arms and legs hasn't occurred to him. In spite of being richly spoiled during the week of vacations he is now again very easy to have. When you are near him he tries to bait you and to divert you to idleness in which he sadly is successful too often. When he is by himself he entertains himself very well. When you hold the jacket for him to get dressed he stretches out his little arms. Because of diarrhea he has to take a grayish powder; now he has become very suspicious and tests every pint or spoonful carefully before he actually starts eating."

That grayish powder for diarrhea was probably mercury, and that could have affected his development. ("Mercury: the gray powder in diarrhea for children," according to the *Merck Manual* from 1905.) We know from our previous work on mercury that acrodynia could provoke neurological symptoms and that mercury containing "grayish powders" weren't recognized as toxic until decades later. Based on this single mention of a possible toxic exposure, it's impossible to know whether P received more mercury exposures than this one. But it's certainly possible that mercury poisoning played a role.

Before the railroad trip, there was little in P's mother's diary that seemed unusual. And for a short time after his mercury exposure, P's development seemed to continue normally for the most part. But early in the second year of life, what Tramer called "the fifth quarter," P appeared to show some abnormal symptoms: "special interest in rhythmic movement," "stereotypical linguistic reaction to something new," and "a vehement rubbing . . . of unusual intensity" of the child's head on his mother. Was this a reaction to mercury in the grayish powder? It's certainly possible.

But it isn't until much later that P's mother reported symptoms that were serious and clear markers of trouble ahead. At two years nine months his mother notes: "Fearful [climbing down from the chair, going down the stairs]. Eats by himself and 'fairly neatly.' Play-peculiarities [turning, twirling]. Toe-walking with strong joyousness. Fierce jealous love, hostility towards children. Obstinacy. Phonographism." At two years ten months: "Autism. Mutism. Phonographism. Dialogue-like talk to himself. Dramatized struggles with conscience." From that point until the end of the diary at four years nine months, there were some ups and downs, but a clearly negative trend. Not surprisingly perhaps, the diary ended when P's course took a decidedly negative turn.

At the end of the paper, Tramer summarized P's symptoms in order to arrive at a diagnosis. "Already early on, as we saw, the total mutism in the form of temporary and elective mutism announced itself. Furthermore we found autism, phonographism, stereotypies, verbigerations, perseverations, blockages, affective perversions, above all others also a remitting course so that at least at first the symptomatological diagnosis of an infantile schizophrenia, a *dementia praecoccissima*, imposes itself."

Not surprisingly, the first candidate for a diagnosis is Heller's syndrome. Tramer wrote that "differential diagnostically [speaking], primarily *dementia infantilis* (Heller) would be under consideration." But the early onset of P's symptoms argues against that. "When we base the essential signs established by Zappert to it, the result is the following: The start of the illness falls already into the 2nd year of life, not just between the 3rd and 4th year as in *dementia infantilis*. Already before that we don't have a completely normal development with P." Tramer concludes, "Because of that we are allowed to exclude a *dementia infantilis*, in spite of individual symptomatological congruences."

After ruling out Heller's, Tramer ends up with a diagnosis that appears little different (remember that De Sanctis's *dementia praecoccissima* and Heller's *dementia infantilis* were not seen as different by most observers). "The diagnostic conclusion that we arrive at after these differential diagnostic considerations accordingly reads as follows: In P.'s case we are probably dealing with an all in all rare case of a genuine early infantile schizophrenia, a *dementia praecoccissima*."

Was P an undiagnosed case of early infantile autism? Or was his odd developmental trajectory a combination of early mercury exposure (the grayish powder at eleven months) and a subsequent onset of *dementia infantilis* (a more typical onset at thirty-three months)? We suspect the latter, but it's certainly possible to read Tramer and conclude otherwise.

◆ ◆ ◆

So ends our search for plausible cases of autism born before 1930, cases with an onset before thirty months and a symptom profile that reasonably matches either Kanner's or Asperger's sentinel cases. In the period from 1890 to 1930, we placed six cases from our collection of ninety-one documented cases inside our Empty Quadrant, possibly making it a little less empty. Of these, at least two (Hellmuth and Don) are probably explained by an early brain injury (birth asphyxia and whooping cough). Another case, P, falls outside the Heller's diagnosis solely due to what might have been a transitory reaction to a mercury treatment. Two of the remaining three, Otto and "Girl," are described only briefly, and the third, Jane, is an arguable case.

If one accepts that these remaining three (Otto, "Girl," and Jane) might reasonably be diagnosed as autistic today, and adds in the three cases from William Howship Dickinson's case notes who were born in the 1870s and the two case descriptions from John Haslam's *Observations on Madness and Melancholia* (both of whom were born in the 1790s and appear to have had adverse vaccine reactions), that gives us a total of eight possible autism cases in a period of 140 years.

Does this mean there might have been scattered cases of autism born before 1930? Yes, quite possibly. Does this place the rate of autism before 1930 above our claim of "effectively zero"? Clearly not. Is Gulliver anywhere in sight? You make the call.

Weygandt Uber Alles

Before we move past 1930 and into the true Age of Autism—where it is no longer necessary to peer into blank spaces with electron microscopes to find cases—we need to finish our tale of Heller-Weygandt with the peculiar future history of the latter, and what it foreshadowed.

Weygandt was a professor in Hamburg. In 1908, the same year Heller published his paper, the same year Hitler came to Vienna from Linz and learned to hate his new home and its polyglot mix of nationalities, artistic styles, and most especially Jews, Weygandt became director of the Hamburg State Hospital and, according to one account, "the most important German authority in the field of research and care" of mentally incapacitated children. That was unfortunate. When Hitler and his long-cultivated hatreds came to power in 1933, Weygandt was quick to apply for membership in the Nazi Party. (He was rejected, apparently for insufficient nationalistic ardor or perhaps because the party, like Theodor Heller a quarter century earlier, smelled an opportunist.) Weygandt was also an enthusiastic eugenicist, believing that most mental illness and criminal behavior was hereditary and that those affected should be prevented from reproducing. He welcomed the Nazi Law for the Prevention of Genetically Diseased Offspring, which advocated for forced sterilization and castration.[93]

Those views underlay the murder ("involuntary euthanasia") of mental defectives in Hitler's "Akton T-4" program that began in 1940; and that program laid the groundwork for the Holocaust. Weygandt was not around to see his ideas reach their logical conclusion; a life-long asthmatic, he died of an attack in 1939, the year after his native land had stolen Austria, where he had himself seen, and stolen, Heller's case of *dementia infantilis*.

Ultimately, the shadow of Hitler and the Nazis played an uncanny role in how autism emerged, spawning claims that Epidemic Deniers have employed to strange effect. The discovery of a new disorder, the battle over priority, the shadow and menace of Nazi ideology—these play out on a much larger stage in the next chapter.

CHAPTER 4

Autism Arrives

"*Tendentious* means promoting a specific, and controversial, point of view. When something is tendentious, it shows a bias towards a particular point of view, especially one that people disagree about. It shares a root with the word, tendency, which means leaning towards acting a certain way."

—Vocabulary.com

A good argument can be made that 1938 was the twentieth century's worst year, and October its absolute nadir. Look at it counterfactually: If Hitler's troops hadn't been allowed to occupy the German-speaking Sudetenland of Czechoslovakia on October 1 against that sovereign country's will, Hitler might not have been lulled into thinking he could go on grabbing territory forever. The carnage that began less than a year later, on September 1, 1939, with the invasion of Poland—followed by England and France's declaration of war that stunned Hitler—might have been foreshortened, or prevented altogether. Instead, events in Munich just about foreordained it.

"Peace in our time," as Chamberlain described the Munich agreement on September 30 (*appeasement* was the word that stuck) gave way to World War II and 50 million deaths, followed by the Cold War and nuclear standoff that enslaved millions more.

The Anschluss—the annexation of Austria in March 1938—was an earlier harbinger. Hitler marched into his native country without resistance and to cheering crowds; Jews were soon jumping from their apartment ledges or being made to clean the streets of Vienna with toothbrushes; Adolf Eichmann took up residence and developed his sick expertise in rounding up and "deporting" them. None of that was quite enough to alert the world to Hitler's sinister designs.

Vienna, capital of Austro-Hungary, where Freud helped create the modern mind, where Heller found his cases, where Popper and Wittgenstein philosophized and Klimt painted his gilded ladies, where Hitler listened to Wagner and seethed at the Jewish immigrants from the East, where Hayek wrote of a liberal world order, was going dark just ahead of the rest of Europe. Jews who survived capture or death had begun fleeing if they could, and many—especially those with professional resumes and someone in the field to sponsor them—resettled in the United States, giving psychiatry a decidedly German Jewish accent for decades to come.

Also in October, a doctor named Hans Asperger, who worked at a children's clinic in Vienna, first spoke publically about an unusual kind of child. His sole use of the term "autistic psychopathy" was buried deep in a paragraph from an obscure three-and-a-half-page speech reprinted in an unremarkable journal, *Wiener Klinische Wochenschrift,* on page 1415.[94]

◆ ◆ ◆

"Since 1938 there have come to our attention . . . "

That fateful October, a child from Forest, Mississippi, named Donald Triplett arrived at the Harriett Lane Home For Invalid Children in Baltimore. The home had a remarkable history.[95] Its namesake, Harriett Rebecca Lane, was born in 1830 in Pennsylvania. Her mother's maiden name was Jane Buchanan. Both parents died by the time she was eleven, and Harriett went to live with her mother's brother, James

Buchanan, an unmarried lawyer from Lancaster, Pennsylvania, who, long story short, was elected president of the United States in 1857. Harriett became the "stiffly formal" president's first lady, a woman of "spontaneity and poise [who] filled the White House with gaiety and flowers" to surround her starched-collar uncle.

When Buchanan left office, she returned with him to Pennsylvania. She married late, at thirty-six, and in the next eighteen years lost her uncle the former president, her husband, and both their sons. Out of this came a bequest to create the Harriett Lane Home for Invalid Children in 1912, on the grounds of Johns Hopkins Hospital in Baltimore—the first home for mentally disturbed children connected to a pediatric treatment center in the United States.

History now intersected in a surprising way with the fury then unfolding in Europe. Leo Kanner, the renowned child psychiatrist at Hopkins, was an Austrian-born Jewish émigré from what is now the Ukraine who came to America well before the Holocaust that claimed most of the Jews in his homeland ("serendipity," he called his early departure, as well as much else to come). In the 1930s, he found himself in position to help other Jewish doctors, and he took full advantage of it, sponsoring more than two hundred to come to the United States.

By 1938, one of the psychiatrists Kanner sponsored had become a member of his staff in Baltimore. His name was Georg Frankl, a Czech by way of Vienna, where he had been, amazingly enough, the chief diagnostician in Hans Asperger's clinic and something of a mentor to the younger man. Frankl married another émigré who had fled the Vienna clinic, Anni Weiss. This link between Asperger's clinic and Kanner was surfaced for the first time by Steve Silberman in *NeuroTribes* and looms large in his argument.

◆ ◆ ◆

At the Harriet Lane Home, Donald was given a quick exam, apparently by Kanner, who dispatched him to the Child Study Home of Maryland, another Hopkins affiliate. According to Kanner, it fell to Frankl and a psychiatrist named Eugenie Cameron to do a more detailed examination over a period of two weeks; their report appears in Kanner's landmark "Autistic Disturbances of Affective Contact" under *Case 1*. Donald T.; Kanner credits their work by name. None of this is disputed.[96]

As a handful of other children with similar behaviors—eight in four years through January 1942, eleven by the time the paper published the next year—arrived in Baltimore, Kanner realized he was seeing a new disorder, one not accounted for in his own comprehensive text on child psychiatry published in 1935. He wrote to Ernest Harms, editor of the new journal *The Nervous Child*, who had asked Kanner to guest-edit an upcoming volume.

"As to the issue due early in 1943, I wonder what you think of the general topic, 'Affective Contact of Children.' I might have paper of my own on 'Autistic Disturbances of Affective Contact in Small Children.' I have followed a number of children who present a very interesting, unique and as yet unreported condition, which has both interested and fascinated me for quite some time. In fact, eventually I plan to use the material for a monographic presentation."[97]

The article appeared in the April 1943 issue under the title "Autistic Disturbances of Affective Contact." It began: "Since 1938 there have come to our attention a number of children whose condition differs so markedly and uniquely from anything reported so far, that each case merits—and, I hope, will eventually receive—a detailed consideration of its fascinating peculiarities.

"*Case 1.* Donald T. was first seen in October, 1938. . . . "

It all seems simple enough.

But the Deniers have picked a fight here over credit and priority for purposes that seem pathetically obvious. Specifically, Silberman in *NeuroTribes* advances the novel claim that Kanner misappropriated the notion of "autistic disturbances of affective contact" from the prior terminology of "autistic psychopathy" that originated with the clinic in Vienna, where Hans Asperger had begun seeing what eventually proved to be a much milder version of "autistic" children (nor was he the first). Silberman proposes a specific mechanism for that misappropriation—that Frankl and Weiss were familiar with autism because they had seen hundreds of cases in Vienna over many years, and they simply told Kanner all about it when they first encountered Donald T. It's a provocative argument and one that's received a lot of attention. However, in order to make his case, Silberman reaches for speculative scenarios and flimsy arguments that far exceed the facts to support them.

Placing Frankl at the center of the autism discovery universe is like putting the earth in the center of the solar system. It has its place, but it's not quite that central. Yet here is Silberman: "If Frankl ever proposed the term Autistischen Psychopathen [used by Asperger] as a name for the boy's condition, Kanner would have likely rejected it out of hand . . . ."[98]

This is some kind of weird claim—that Kanner might have rejected a term that we have no knowledge Frankl might have proposed. Or this, on Kanner's alleged vast but illicit debt to Asperger via Frankl: "This crucial link [Frankl's role] between the two pioneers of autism has escaped the attention of historians until now, mostly because Kanner studiously avoided mentioning it. He never acknowledged Asperger's contributions to the field—a fact that has puzzled autism scholars for decades."[99]

You don't say. We found a March 26, 1971, letter from Kanner to D. Arn van Krevelen commending him for writing a paper on autism and Asperger's that "fulfills a most significant purpose—the one about which we originally corresponded—namely after about three decades to make the American 'experts' aware that Asperger did not 'copy from,' 'confirm,' 'agree with' me. You have no idea how many people here have ever heard of Asperger." This is not the voice of a man who has been ducking any acknowledgement of Asperger for as long as humanly possible.

Fortunately, Kanner said, van Krevelen had fashioned "a masterful, clearly expressed, indisputable juxtaposition of the distinguishing features of early infantile autism and autistic psychopathy [the English version of the phrase Silberman says he would have rejected out of hand if Frankl had mentioned it!]. It had to be brought to the attention of the American reader, and, as I anticipated, could not be set down so lucidly and succinctly by anybody else, not even by myself or by Asperger." (The chart we reproduce at the end of the next chapter is from that paper.)

But Silberman sees glory hogging everywhere: "[Kanner's] unpublished memoir, written in the 1950s, names Frankl as one of many clinicians whom he helped immigrate to America in the years leading up to the war but comes to a mysteriously abrupt end just before the breakthrough that made him famous. Kanner's colleagues maintained that he was simply unfamiliar with the parallel work unfolding in Vienna at the time, and he never corrected them."[100]

Now this is really reaching. Kanner foreshortened his autobiography, "mysteriously" ending just short of autism, to avoid crediting Frankl? Good grief. Well, we saw the last pages of the manuscript at Kanner's son's Albert's home in Madison, Wisconsin, in 2009, and they were few and, frankly, uninteresting, given everything that had already been written on the topic, including by Kanner himself. Kanner never found a publisher for the autobiography. We read it, and we see why. One editor whose letter is preserved in Kanner's archive politely noted that he devoted way too many pages to his early years in Europe (picaresque though they were, including a rousing account of losing his virginity). Kanner the autobiographer may simply have run out of anecdotes and gas. It happens; why would anyone assume instead that Kanner's failure to finish was to keep Frankl, the all-knowing arbiter of autism, in the shadows?

Furthermore, Donald T., the child that Kanner credits for his own "Eureka!" moment of discovery, was not in fact the first such child seen at the clinic. A boy known as Alfred L. from Baltimore was referred to Hopkins in November of 1935, two years before Frankl arrived.[101] Yet Silberman suggests *Frankl*, like Mighty Mouse come to save the day for the yokels at Hopkins, is responsible for even this connection: "Shortly after [Donald T.'s father's] letter arrived from Mississippi, someone in his [Kanner's] office asked the mother of a boy called Alfred L., who had been seen at the clinic back in 1935, for an update on her son's development. Was Frankl digging through old files, looking for similar cases that had fallen through the cracks?"[102]

No, he was bloody well not. Isn't it 100 percent more likely the person digging through old files was Leo Kanner himself or someone he deputized, or someone else who had been on the Hopkins staff in 1935 and *remembered* Alfred L., for heaven's sake, not someone like Frankl who was back in Vienna writing about how people talk to dogs?

Well, isn't it?

Against Silberman's bizarre elevation of Frankl (and, it must be said, sliming of Kanner) should be weighed the small matters of Kanner saving Frankl's life and that of his future wife, promoting his success in academia, and giving him one of the few publication credits of his entire career by running an article next to Kanner's in *The Nervous Child*. Nonetheless, Kanner "exploited" Frankl for his own nefarious purposes? This is where the story stood when *NeuroTribes* made its splash January 16, 2014, with Frankl front and center: like Wilhelm Weygandt before him, Kanner had hijacked an important diagnosis, made it his own, and screwed things up for everyone.

Silberman: "In real world terms being locked out of a diagnosis often meant being denied access to education, speech and occupational therapy, counseling, medication, and other forms of support. For undiagnosed adults, Kanner's insistence that autism was a disorder of early infancy meant decades of wandering in the wilderness with no explanation for constant struggles in employment, dating, friendships and simply navigating the chaos of daily life."[103]

◆ ◆ ◆

To regain our bearings, let's look at Frankl's piece that ran alongside Kanner's in that issue of *The Nervous Child*. Titled "Language and Affective Contact,"[104] Frankl's article took up the case of a boy named Karl K., whose failure to communicate in any fashion made him stand out among other cases—post encephalitic Parkinson's, deaf-mute, aphasic, word blind. Frankl distinguishes between deficits of word language and emotional language and contrasts Karl K.'s severe deficits in both areas with cases (including emotionally intelligent dogs!) having deficits in only one. "He neither received nor sent out any communicative symbols. This is a most impressive phenomenon: a boy who undoubtedly sees and hears, does not take any notice of a person who clearly and conspicuously enters the field of his senses and addresses him."

In a comment that echoes features of autism, Frankl wrote, "His attitude toward the children and also toward the adults around him was similar to the attitude healthy persons assume toward the objects in their environment. They use them, but they don't communicate with them or expect reciprocity."

But there were other features of Karl K.'s profile that have greater relevance to his behavior and lack of "affective contact." Most notably, he was severely mentally retarded, or as Frankl put it, "he was imbecile." Frankl described him as "a sturdy well-built boy with primitive facial features and dull expression . . . he did not speak at all. Never in his life had he said a word or uttered a sound."

There was little mystery about the source of Karl's disability. He had tuberous sclerosis, a rare genetic illness that causes benign tumors to spread throughout the body. Half of those with the disorder have learning difficulties. Somewhere between a quarter and a third meet the criteria for autism, while others fit the broader category of pervasive developmental disorders.

In this we are reminded of earlier cases cited by Down, which we believe may have been Fragile X syndrome, another risk factor for autism.

So this child, born around 1930 and profiled in a psychiatric publication edited by Leo Kanner, had a predisposing genetic vulnerability to autism. Clearly, the article was paired with Kanner's because the child had a profound disorder of affective contact; it did not belong in Kanner's article directly—his children were otherwise typical—but it also treated affective contact as an important theme. How this amounts to shunting Frankl off to the side or denying him the chance to address the topic is beyond us.

A stark example of Silberman's tendentiousness is his account of Frankl's sole manuscript addressed to autism in childhood. In 1957, Frankl, by then director of the Child Guidance Clinic at the University of Kansas, wrote a sixty-two-page monograph.[105] Apparently, it was never published and now sits in an archive at the university. In this manuscript, Frankl describes nine cases of severely autistic children, makes mention neither of his experience in Vienna nor of Hans Asperger, and compliments Kanner on his "initial, excellent, though summary descriptions of early infantile autism." There is no hint of residual jealousy, simply a great deal of theorizing about the nature of the autistic "state of mind" and the use of language in these nine severe cases, long a fascination of Frankl's.

Buried deeply in the draft—page forty-three of sixty-two—Frankl makes a glancing reference to the variability of language skills in autistic children: "A continuum seems to stretch out between the two extremes, with Johnny of case 1 as representative of the one extreme; the intellectually superior schizoid child as representative of the other. We know of this continuum and we can point out a few of its common characteristics and a few symptoms characteristic for some phases in this continuum."

In his thorough review of Frankl's role in the history of autism, a well-known scholar with Asperger's syndrome, John Robison, cites this manuscript, noting that Frankl "had written of a continuum but made little of the idea."[106] But Silberman takes this obscure 1957 passage and magnifies it beyond all reason. He misrepresents Frankl's glancing reference to a "continuum" as further evidence of "what had been forgotten in the endless debates about clinical nomenclature." He claims, erroneously, that Frankl illustrated this continuum with three case descriptions. In fact, none of the nine cases Frankl describes bear any resemblance to Asperger's Little Professors. All were readily identifiable as severe Kanner-type autism; one might have been a case of *dementia infantilis*.

Silberman, however, is unconstrained by such prosaic facts. He inflates references in Frankl's paper to "a child prodigy" and "a schizoid genius" as evidence Frankl conceptualized the notion of an autism spectrum that Lorna Wing later elaborated.[107] If not entirely false, it's a gross exaggeration of Frankl's argument and a misrepresentation of his evidence; in fact, "the intellectually superior schizoid child" Silberman sets up at one end of Frankl's supposed continuum is not even given as a case history in the paper. There is no "schizoid genius" or "child prodigy" cited outside of that glancing reference.

After seeing the citations of this 1957 paper in both *NeuroTribes* and Robison's review, we found Frankl's original document and read it with interest. If Silberman were right and Frankl were indeed the true pioneer in discovering the autism spectrum, certainly his sole surviving discussion of "autism in childhood" would provide evidence for his historic role. We can imagine Silberman's sense of anticipation as he first opened the document. We can imagine no other reaction, after reading it, than deflation. Nothing in the text shows Frankl writing about the "lost tribe" of Hans Asperger; instead, he was clearly following in the tradition of Leo Kanner, with descriptions of a severely impaired childhood population.

The final blow to Silberman's speculative excesses came five months after publication of his own book, when Donvan and Zucker's *In a Different Key* was published. Those authors actually obtained Donald's medical records—for which they deserve not just credit but our thanks.

In the space for diagnosis, the medical team, presumably Frankl and Cameron, wrote two words—*Heller's,* and *Schizophrenia*—with a question mark at the beginning.

? Heller's Schizophrenia

"The rest of the space," Donvan and Zucker note, "was blank."[108] There is no evidence that Frankl, as a primary diagnostician, offered any input at any point on any disorder that was anything like Asperger's. Instead, the bafflement appeared universal. "Judging by their notes, the examining team was thoroughly startled and confused by what they were seeing," Zucker and Donvan wrote.

Bam! This new evidence renders Silberman's "Kanner stole it" theory retrospectively dead on arrival, not that it had much to recommend it in the first place. Silberman's core claim—that Kanner's misappropriation and mischaracterization of Asperger's "lost tribe" condemned generations of gifted humans to a life of misunderstanding and unfulfilled potential—was shattered.

◆ ◆ ◆

Throughout his book, Silberman weaves a seductive web of plausible arguments and titillating facts, but the critical evidence on which he bases his argument collapses under close inspection—and not just by us, as Donvan and Zucker's important finding show. Could anything more clearly demonstrate the blank space (we called it The Empty Quadrant) before 1930 than the questioning and surprise with which Donald T. was greeted? Qualified observers were for the first time seeing a disorder never before described. Their only available diagnostic labels were Heller's and childhood schizophrenia, just as we've argued. No mention of Asperger's "autistic psychopathy."

This sequence of surprise leading to the discovery of a new diagnosis is not that complicated unless one wants it to be. Epidemic Deniers want it to be.

◆ ◆ ◆

Four years later, after Mary Triplett wrote Kanner to suggest that he in fact knew Donald's diagnosis but was sparing them the news, Kanner acknowledged: "At no time have you or your husband been given a clear-cut and unequivocal evaluation in the sense of a diagnostic term." Kanner told Mary that he had "come to recognize for the first time a condition which has not hitherto been described by psychiatric or any other literature."[109]

Once again, Kanner calls the disorder new and different. Is there a Denier alive who is simply willing to take him at his repeated word, soon to be corroborated by a whole community of child psychiatrists? Epidemic Denial is such a convenient argument that its flimsy foundations are ignored even by academics and researchers of repute. Such is the case with this fawning review *of NeuroTribes* by Simon Baron-Cohen, professor of developmental psychopathology at Cambridge, the second oldest university in the English-speaking world, in the *Spectator,* the oldest continuously published magazine in English:[110]

"Steve Silberman's stunning new book looks across history, back to Henry Cavendish, the 18th-century natural scientist who discovered hydrogen, Hugo Gernsbach, the early-20th-century inventor and pioneer of amateur 'wireless' radio, and countless other technically brilliant but socially awkward, eccentric non-conformists, members of the 'neurotribe' we now call the autism spectrum."

Not so. But as to Kanner and Frankl, Baron-Cohen writes: "Silberman also finds something altogether more disturbing: a man who was desperate to make his name in the history of medicine, and who seemed to have been willing to do some rather underhanded things to achieve this goal.

Far from finding Kanner to be a man who was unaware that some 4,000 miles away in Vienna, struggling under Nazi occupation, a fellow physician had described a similar group of patients, Silberman unearths evidence that Kanner must have known about Asperger's work. How? Because Georg Frankl, the chief diagnostician in Asperger's clinic in 1938, came to Johns Hopkins University to work in Kanner's clinic later that year. Long before the Internet or email, the transmission of scientific ideas could nevertheless flow from one lab to another through a doctor working in both. Frankl had crossed the Atlantic and Silberman's argument is that Kanner heard about these special children in Vienna, found some similar ones in his Baltimore clinic, and repackaged them as his own discovery.

Yes, that's his argument, all right, tendentiously flogging a theory for which there is simply no good evidence. Donvan and Zucker saw *NeuroTribes* in time to add a footnote: "As this book was nearing publication, journalist Steve Silberman published his book *NeuroTribes*. In it he reported his original finding that a Czech diagnostician named Georg Frankl, who worked under Kanner in Baltimore in this period, had previously worked alongside the Austrian pediatrician Hans Asperger in Vienna. Silberman contends that through Frankl, and through Kanner's own reading of German-language medical journals, Kanner would have known that Asperger had already used the term autistic as early as 1938. We find Silberman's discovery of Frankl's connection to both men intriguing. Moreover, his theory that Kanner built aspects of Asperger's thinking into his own model of autism, without crediting him, cannot be ruled out as a possibility. However, it seems just as plausible that Kanner, like Asperger, borrowed the term autistic from Swiss psychiatrist Eugen Bleuler, who famously used it in 1911. . . . "[111]

It is galling to read supposition after supposition from Silberman, culminating in Kanner supposedly consigning his colleagues to the dustbin of history: "Kanner seemed resistant to ceding an inch of his authority to his Viennese counterparts, even if it meant confining his former assistant [Frankl] to historical oblivion."

Memo to would-be historians of medicine: watch out for large claims based on events that "seemed" likely, ideas that are "intriguing," scenarios that have "possibility" and "plausibility," and caveats such as "must have known," "could," "intellectual theft—if true," and unadorned calumnies like "underhanded," and "additional acts that Kanner *was also guilty of.*" (Italics ours.)

Baron-Cohen seems almost giddy with gratitude to find a lengthy and popular book endorsing his own wild speculation about "assortative mating" and geek genes. Here we see the Denier matrix suck the brains out of otherwise reasonable people and use them to energize dumb ideas.

◆ ◆ ◆

"Little Professors"

While autism arrived in Baltimore with a bang, what we now call Asperger's crept into Europe on little cat feet. There is convincing evidence of Little Professor syndrome as a rare but real phenomenon before Hans Asperger made his name with it in 1944.

Almost two decades before, in 1926, a Russian researcher, G. E. Sukhareva, wrote a paper called "Schizoid Personality Disorders of Childhood."[112] While "schizoid" may suggest severe mental illness, in Sukhareva's hands it became part of a label for children who had problems that were not necessarily debilitating: *diagnosis: personality disorder: schizoid (eccentric)."* Her cases were born between 1909 and 1914.

The 1996 translation by S. Wolff is titled "The First Account of the Syndrome Asperger Described," and begins, "On reading the paper which follows, it will at once be clear that the six boys described by Dr. Sukhareva some 70 years ago resemble very closely the children reported on by Asperger in 1944 and those more recently described by other workers."

Sukhareva notes, as have so many of the qualified investigators we've quoted, that "childhood personality disorders are relatively rarely described in the literature" but that the six boys between two and fourteen that were referred to her over the previous three years create an interesting cluster.

Case 1, then thirteen years old, "aroused parental anxiety from early childhood because he was different from other children. Even in his crib he was unusually sensitive, particularly to noise, startling at every sound . . . shy, easily frightened and suspicious, he shunned the company of other children. . . . Compliant, quiet, and passive, he initiated no independent activity," instead wandering aimlessly, "bemused at times, and puts numerous absurd questions to the people around him. He repeats these over and over until he gets a comprehensive reply."

He was also precocious, reading at age four and gifted musically. He was accepted by the Conservatoire's school for stringed instruments. But his obsessions and inability to concentrate overcame his gifts and in 1924, he was admitted to Sukhareva's hospital-school. Upon examination, he was found to have tic-like movements, rapid but unclear speech, and an uncanny ability to define words (beauty is "the appearance of

76

an object in a form that is pleasing to the eye"; the difference between obstinacy and persistence is that "the obstinate person acts without reason; the persistent person as a matter of principle'). The doctor's summary: "High artistic gifts in the presence of overall impairment."

The other cases followed suit: Case 2 learned to read at five "and read avidly whatever came to hand," but at school was "severely maladjusted" and never followed rules, engaging in "senseless, impulsive behavior." "Argues a lot; talks a great deal in a stereotyped way, always about the same topic: the War of 1812. A compulsive element is evident in his discourse; if interrupted, he becomes agitated, waits for a convenient moment and then starts his tale all over again, from the beginning and in minute detail."

Case 3: Even at five years his parents found him a "strange" child. "Periodically he developed strong interests and then pursued them exclusively"; at six, he began doing extensive mathematical calculations but dropped it entirely after three months."

Case 6 was described as "a reserved, silent 'little old man,' with an urge to seek solitude and quietness in order to withdraw into his inner world."

"In all our cases schizoid features began in early childhood," wrote Sukhareva. "In most of our cases environmental causes could be excluded on the basis of a detailed case history; pathogenic factors such as brain pathology, intoxication, or a poor child rearing environment were absent. Furthermore, the symptoms had been persistently present since early childhood."

What are we to make of this distinctive cluster of "eccentric" children that now seem like harbingers of Asperger's children? Had they been around forever—the Epidemic Denial argument as applied specifically to Asperger's? That seems unlikely; Sukhareva notes "there have been no previous descriptions of schizoid personality disorder [her name for the syndrome] in children," although she cites a scattering of cases of people with schizoid personality disorder, all over sixteen. "All these patients had manifested autism [in the sense of extreme self-absorption], negativistic tendencies and frequent hebephrenic or catatonic outbursts since early childhood." A scattering of cases does not an epidemic make.

She continued: "Our observations force us to conclude that there is a group of personality disorders whose clinical picture shares certain features with schizophrenia, but which yet differ profoundly from schizophrenia in terms of pathogenesis."

◆ ◆ ◆

Asperger's could just as easily have been called "Sukhareva's" were it not for the historical happenstance of time and place and nomenclature. Asperger's paper was nearly coincident with Kanner's and used "autistic" as Kanner did. But Asperger was, in truth, not even second in line to describe a Little Professor. In 1935, in Vienna, Anni B. Weiss wrote a paper about how to test the intelligence of "psychopathic children,"[113] based on expertise gathered "due to the experience gained from many years work"; Weiss's ideas on testing such children are not remembered, but the detailed description she gave of one such child reads very much like Sukhareva.

"Gottfried K., nine and one-half years of age, was brought for examination by his grandmother on account of difficulties in his upbringing that followed from his extreme nervousness and his queer and helpless behavior in his intercourse with other children" Weiss wrote. "At first sight, the examiner took him for a feebleminded child. But the grandmother's report as well as the child's success at school were inconsistent with that." So Gottfried was kept for four weeks at the children's clinic. He was afraid of children, "even younger ones," as well as dogs, darkness, loud noises, the wind, clouds, and many other nameless terrors. He was clumsy and helpless, cheerful and childish; the other kids laughed at him and called him the "fool."

Weiss proved an insightful and empathic observer. "So we find him absolutely dependent on guidance from the outside, lacking initiative of his own, and we must ask: What does he really feel his position in his environment to be? What are his personal reactions to his surroundings? . . . His own position in the social group or his wishes were never even hinted at in his accounts. Superficial observers might think perhaps he had given up trying to make a place for himself in the group because he had so often been teased. 'They always call me a fool,' he once said to the observer, quite objectively, seeming not to be angry, sorry, or ashamed, and speaking in the rather precocious manner in which he used to recount the naughtiness of other children."

Although they didn't yet realize it—Gottfried was at that point a sample of 1—the Little Professor phenotype had arrived in Austria. Weiss labeled Gottfried with the broad term commonly in use at the Vienna clinic, a "psychopathic child," interesting enough to be mentioned in twenty of the twenty-six pages of the paper. He showed a peculiar and unique profile in his intelligence testing.

Choosing the word "psychopathy" to describe a child is an interesting decision; it first was used in a criminal context in Russia in the 1880s, when a confessed murderer was freed on the grounds that he was a psychopath, presumably unable to control his antisocial behavior. The Oxford English Dictionary says a psychopath is a "mentally ill person who is highly irresponsible and antisocial and also violent or aggressive."

Unlike Sukhareva, Weiss made no claim that this was the first such child to be described; nor did Asperger when he described a similar case in 1938 speech. What Asperger did do uniquely was couple the word "psychopathy" with "autistic"—Bleuler's schizophrenic descriptor.

The phrase *autistic psychopathy* was the label that stuck for the Little Professors—it became Asperger's discovery and claim to fame. "Autism" at that point wasn't sufficient as a label because it was just a symptom of schizophrenia; psychopathy itself was not sufficient because it described a broader set of kids—problem children with all kinds of antisocial behavior.

There's little reason to get excited about psychopathy as another place to look for Gulliver, our mascot for the supposed "hidden horde" of overlooked autistic children. We can find no evidence of autism in contemporaneous description of psychopathic children outside of Anni Weiss. In 1938, Asperger uses the combination phrase for the first time, and, as with Sukhareva, is beginning to say there might be a pattern, but the suggestion is made in only a single paragraph deep in a longer speech. Asperger described only two cases there; in his 1944 paper he only gave case histories of four.

The key paragraph from his 1938 speech is as follows:

Within this well-defined group of children, whom we, because of the constraints of their relationship to their environment, and because of the limits to the own self (αὐτός), call "autistic psychopaths" [autistische Psychopathen], there are again a good number of people who have to be evaluated quite differently. On the one hand the originality of thinking (a little bit of autism always belongs to that!) or the intensity of the specialized interests, which apparently are 'hypertrophied' at the price of [losing] many other abilities, stand in such a way in the foreground that they are capable of producing achievements of the highest quality (who doesn't know the autistic explorer, who, because of his ineptitude and lack of instinct has become a cartoon character, but who, at the same time, can achieve outstanding results or at least advance his narrow special area of expertise!). Another time autistic originality shows up only as wrong-headed, cranky, and useless (that a direction of a thought is felt as unusual and peculiar may have its basis in the fact that it points to the future and can, at a later date, become living reality, or instead doesn't have anything at all to do with reality). In this last mentioned group of autistic psychopaths, then, the disturbed ability to adapt to the environment, the inability to learn, stands in the foreground, and determines the social prognosis in an unfavorable sense. From such pictures of greatly disturbed personalities, there may be fluent transitions to schizophrenia, the essential symptom of which is also indeed autism, the loss of any contact with the environment. The connection of such pictures to schizophrenia is also seen in the fact that you can find among the relatives of such people not merely autistic eccentrics but also greater quantities of real schizophrenics.[114]

It would not be until six years later that Asperger describes his larger group, still only four children but enough to attach his name to the disorder. The paper was called "Autistic Psychopathy in Childhood." In the introduction he continued his exploration that he began as a brief tangent in his 1938 speech. A lengthy introduction to his 1944 paper (one which no one has bothered to translate in print, considering its excessive throat clearing) describes in some depth the intellectual context in which he was working. In turgid doctoral prose, he describes different systems for deviance and personality, citing several authors who had dealt with the problem of psychopathy and how to describe and classify it. It is clear he viewed his selection of Little Professors as another variant, a subtle and fascinating one, of what the clinic called "psychopathy," what some might simply call juvenile delinquency today. Asperger wrote the following:

> In the following a type of children is being described which seems in many ways worthy of interest: A uniform basic distur- bance that quite typically expresses itself in the physical, in the appearances of expression, in the whole behavior, determines . . . characteristic difficulties in adaptability; . . . again in other cases there is compensation through special originality of thinking and experiencing that often also lead to special performance in later life. The demand that special persons who . . . also needed special pedagogical treatment that is adapted to their special difficulties can be well documented with these psychopaths. And finally here it can also be shown that deviant persons, too, are able to fulfill their place in the framework of the larger social community, par- ticularly when they find understanding, loving leadership.[115]

These cases, as novel as they appeared, are not marked by the disability or presence from the beginning of life as seen in Kanner's contempo- raneous cases. They are considered as one more variant of the devi- ant caseload normally seen by Frankl, Weiss, and Asperger, and their unique flavor of deviance simply provides another opportunity for edu- cational innovation to set them on a path toward rehabilitation. By con- trast, none of the eleven Kanner children would have been visualized making outstanding contributions in a particular field of expertise.

And none of Asperger's "psychopaths" had the same sharply defined onset at birth or in infancy. As Arn van Krevelen remarked later, "The manifestation age of autistic psychopathy is in the first years of elementary school, or earlier if the parents have not been able to adjust themselves to the individualistic behavior of their child. Never is the diagnosis made in infancy."[116] In Kanner's autism, of course, the diagnosis was *always* evident from infancy, which sim- ply demonstrates the deep differences in the conditions despite their superficial kinship.

◆ ◆ ◆

For our purposes here there are two important issues: when were these children born and how many of them were there?

Sukhareva's cases were born around 1910. Gottfried was in the early 1920s; Asperger's two cases from his speech may well have been born before 1930; and as we've said before only one of the four in his 1944 paper was born before 1930 and that was Hellmuth, who probably didn't fit the pattern. (The small number of cases in his series is notable given that most such contemporary reports of Heller-Weygandt or childhood schizophrenia used far more to make their point; Kanner had eleven; Lay and Sukhareva had six; Heller had six in 1908. One gets the feeling Weiss and Asperger were reporting on all the cases they had seen, not on a judicious selection designed to highlight different traits.)

So we can find scattered cases of Little Professors before 1930, scattered in enough quantity that they were described as a group before then as well. But they were only described in two parts of the world, Moscow and Vienna, and generally as unique in some fashion. So we think it's fair to assume they were not present in large numbers. Oddly, the Epidemic Deniers have used these few case reports to make the argument that "Asperger's Lost Tribe" had simply been overlooked. They are supported in this not by Sukhareva or Weiss but by Asperger, who, in his 1938 speech, describes his two Little Professors as evidence of a larger category of children, and in 1944 said, "We want only to state briefly that over the course of 10 years we have observed more than 200 children who all showed autism to a greater or lesser degree."

How are we to make sense of this claim of a far larger number of cases than are supported by any evidence? We think that has more to do with the moment in history we've described at the start of the chapter. A Viennese clinic for problem children in the early 1930s run largely by Jews was one of the most vulnerable settings one could possibly imagine. The particular circumstances of "The Heilpedagogical Station of the Children's Clinic at the University of Vienna"[117] demand closer inspection.

A Clinic in Crisis

The true history of the Vienna clinic is becoming wrapped up in the agenda of Epidemic Deniers. In Silberman's telling, it was an island of compassion and healing pedagogy in a world blind to the suffering of the brilliant Little Professors, misunderstood children who were invisible to the world. In Silberman's dramatis personae, Asperger is the inspirational leader, his Jewish colleagues Anni Weiss and Georg Frankl the true discoverers of autism, and Kanner just an interloper who skewed the story of the discovery of autism to his own interest.

In this telling, Frankl, Weiss, and Asperger were the beneficiaries of the vision of Erwin Lazar, who started the university clinic in Vienna, the first of its kind, and taught them to treat every child as a whole being, not as a subject of scientific inspection.

Is this really the truth or just the rewriting of a more mundane history? There's a far more straightforward view of the clinic Asperger came to lead. In 1911, Lazar, who had been a student of the great Bleuler (who coined the word autism that same year), was appointed the first leader of the "therapeutical pedagogical station" at the students' clinic at the University of Vienna.

His initial focus was on troubled children, working with the juvenile court system and schools. He wrote articles on criminology and family dynamics, truancy, and childhood suicide. In modern parlance, one might speak of the "therapeutical pedagogical station" as a juvenile detention or correction center. A 1935 observer described the clinic as concerned with "neglected, delinquent, neuropathic, psychopathic and feeble-minded children" who were referred "from special institutions, juvenile courts, schools and private sources." There were twenty-one beds; the children, age one and a half to seventeen years of age, were up at six o'clock and into bed at seven-thirty; the average stay was four to six weeks."[118]

Under Lazar's leadership, there was a small staff: Weiss, Frankl, Joseph Feldner, and Sister Viktorine, a nun. Hans Asperger joined the staff upon Lazar's death in 1932.

There is little to suggest anything especially remarkable about any of these professionals; Lazar was, by far, the most prolific writer but leaves no record of interest in autistic psychopathy; Frankl and Weiss wrote a handful of articles including Weiss's description of Gottfried, which evinced less interest in his unique profile and more in her IQ testing methods.

Frankl wrote an article in 1933 titled, "Ordering and Obeying,"[119] perhaps influenced by the obstreperous youth that confronted him every morning at 6:00 a.m. (For a man Silberman describes as a pioneer of "neurodiversity" and one of the world's great humanitarians, Frankl had an odd preoccupation with obedience.) Far from foreshadowing "Asperger's lost tribe," Frankl's deservedly obscure paper was a lengthy exegesis on the notion that what one says is heard differently depending on how one says it. A decade later, he would write the aforementioned article on "language and affective contact" alongside Kanner, and a decade after that, an unpublished manuscript on autism. Was Frankl a dedicated and caring man? We have no reason to believe otherwise. But was he the unsung hero of autism? There is no evidence of any kind that indicates in any way that he was exceptional.

In fact, the Vienna clinic's entire orientation—its emphasis on psychopathy in children, Frankl's interest in the role of language and gesture in "ordering and obeying," and Weiss's mechanical interest in the way intelligence testing methods could be used to improve teaching methods targeted at their psychopathic caseload—gives the whole place the flavor of what generations of Americans might call "juvie hall," where young miscreants are sent to reform before turning into hardened criminals beyond the beneficent but Teutonic reach of the Heilpedagogical Station regimen.

◆ ◆ ◆

By the early 1930s, the winds of change were blowing. Anti-Semitism was rising in places like Austria. According to a recent historical review by John Robison in the journal *Autism,* Weiss was dismissed in the fall of 1934 and Frankl left in late 1937. The hospital leadership had recently changed with the 1930 appointment of Franz Hamburger. He reportedly had antisemitic views and was also the mentor and thesis adviser for Hans Asperger.

In the United States, Kanner was doing his best to help European Jews escape the looming Nazi threat. Anni Weiss, who by that time had made her way to the United States, was able to influence Kanner to bring Frankl over. Frankl arrived just in time to have Kanner assign him to evaluate Donald T.

Silberman uses all this as he tries to knock down Kanner's priority in the discovery of autism. Donvan and Zucker go after Asperger with a far harsher claim: he was a Nazi sympathizer, or at least a gutless enabler, who sent disabled children to their deaths. Silberman's hero becomes Donvan and Zucker's villain, and vice versa, both extremes fulfilling a respective purpose—Silberman slams Kanner for suppressing the "lost tribe" Asperger championed, while Donvan and Zucker go after Asperger for embodying the inhumane treatment that people with autism and their families endured for decades. (These are flavors two and three of autism denial from the introduction.)

On October 3 of that critical year, the month Donald T. arrived in Baltimore and met Asperger's former colleague Frankl, Asperger gave a speech titled "The Psychology of the Abnormal Child"[120] that began with praise for the new order.

"We are right in the middle of a mighty remodeling project of our life that has gripped all areas of this life, not the least the medical profession. The overriding thought of the new empire: The whole is more than its parts. The people are more important than the individual." He acknowledged the "effort to prevent the passing on of pathological genetic traits—in very many cases that belong here we are dealing with heritable disturbances—and to promote the traits that are genetically healthy. We physicians have to submit with full responsibility to those tasks that arise particularly in this area."

Whatever the motive—to make a perfunctory bow in hopes of being left alone, or as a craven attempt to curry favor—the words evoke an era when "the best lack all conviction and the worst are full of passionate intensity." (Yeats, *Slouching Toward Bethlehem,* on the aftermath of World War I.) But then his talk took on a different tone, with a discussion of "abnormal children" and "how much can we accomplish for these human beings?" The answer: quite a lot. "When we help them with all our devotion, we are also performing the best service for our people; not only by keeping them from burdening society as a whole through their anti-social and criminal acts, but also in that we are trying to achieve that they will occupy their place as working human beings in the living organism of the people."

Don't kill them, seemed to be the subtext; *put them to work* in the new world order.

Asperger, it quickly becomes clear, was singling out a group of high-functioning individuals as opposed to intellectually disabled or mentally ill children; Weiss's paper highlighting Gottfried from 1935 immediately suggests itself. He starts with the case of a ten-year-old boy referred to his outpatient clinic.

"He is in the first grade of middle school. The father reports horrible difficulties. In the foreground is his sensitivity not only in the physical realm (in several sensory areas), but above all his psychological sensitivity.

"Here are several examples: There are from the beginning great difficulties with eating. He does not like all kinds of foods. Instead of that he passionately loves strongly sour things (by the way, we find this trait often in psychopathic children). He has difficulties falling asleep particularly when there is unrest around him or when he has eaten too short a time before going to bed. All in all his sleep is too light.

"He is very anxious and insecure, and fears at all kinds of occasions for his health. Trivialities he takes very much to heart, is sometimes, as he says himself, 'quite melancholic.' The greatest conflicts, however, come from his psychological sensitivity, his irritability: From the smallest occurrence result scenes in which he 'behaves as if he was crazy.' The father then also comes with the question whether the boy is psychologically normal."

He is, Asperger says, "constant at the limits of his self-control in an only little bit unusual situation." But that's just half the story, Asperger says. "The boy has another side, which, seemingly, stands in strange contrast to the described abnormal symptoms. He is far above his age in intelligence. Indicative for that is his language that, with the complicated sentence structure and choice of words absolutely compares to the language of a grown-up. He poses himself religious and philosophical problems, observes people from a genuine psychological interest and has a good eye for their peculiarities, particularly their weaknesses. It is understood that he has always been first in his class, that his essays 'are called out as sensational,' that he does not make orthographic mistakes, that he easily passed the entrance exam to middle school.

"To summarize the diagnosis: We are dealing with an intellectually particularly gifted, character-wise finely differentiated, delicately sensitive boy with numerous physical and psychological sensitivities."

Addressing Asperger's speech, Donvan and Zucker wrote, "His salute to the Anschluss, to the Nazis, to the suppression of individuality, and to the task of purifying the genetic lineage of the nation should by itself have dealt a fatal blow to the idea that Asperger secretly resisted the Nazi agenda." They continue, "A review of other medical talks and papers printed that year in the same weekly journal where Asperger's appeared shows that the opening of his talk was far from typical. Defenders of Asperger sometimes argue that he had a hidden anti-Nazi agenda—that he sought to throw the Gestapo off his scent by paying lip service to the regime. Brita Schirmer described the preamble as a 'deft chess move' on Asperger's part. His defenders usually assert, as a corollary, that the full text of Asperger's speech, together with his 1944 paper, constitute an unambiguous argument to protect and nurture all vulnerable children, no matter the level of their disability."[121]

Adam Feinstein's *A History of Autism* believes the text shows a doctor trying to throw the Nazis off the trail—and barely succeeding. "The Gestapo came twice to Asperger's Clinic to arrest him and was protected on both occasions by Hamburger," whose loyalty to his mentee appeared to overtake his Nazi sympathies.[122]

Feinstein quotes from a 1974 radio interview with Asperger:

In Heilpadagogik, we had a great deal of contact with disturbed, mentally deficient children. We had no choice to but recognize their value and love them. What is their value? They belong to the population, they are indispensable for some jobs but also for the ethos which teaches us how we humans are committed to one another. It is totally inhuman—as we saw with dreadful consequences—when people accept the concept of a worthless life. . . . As I was never willing to accept this concept—in other words, to notify the [Nazi] Health Office of the mentally deficient [children in my charge]—this was truly a dangerous situation for me. I just give great credit to my mentor Hamburger, because although he was a convinced National Socialist, he saved me twice from the Gestapo with strong, personal commitment. He knew my attitude but he protected me with his whole being, and for that I have the greatest appreciation.

Clearly, although Zucker and Donvan recognize the pro-Asperger argument, they aren't buying it. They go on to describe a letter Asperger wrote in 1941, unearthed recently by a researcher, Herwig

Czech, and presented to a colloquium on Asperger in a talk titled, "Dr. Hans Asperger and the Nazi Child Euthanasia Program in Vienna: Possible Connections." Czech found the letter in the archives of the Spiegelgrund—described by Donvan and Zucker as "the facility on Vienna's outskirts which superficially resembled a hospital, but which functioned in reality as a killing center for severely disabled children. Those chosen for death at the Spiegelgrund were poisoned by phenobarbital, which was administered in suppositories, or mixed into the children's meals. The drug, in sufficient doses, causes the lungs to malfunction. As a rule, 'pneumonia' was listed as the official cause of death."[123]

Asperger's letter described a two-year-old girl named Herta Schreiber who contracted encephalitis and was now brain damaged. In his own handwriting, Asperger told the hospital's administration: "When at home, this child must present an unbearable burden to the mother, who has to care for five healthy children." He recommended "permanent placement" at the facility, which Donvan and Zucker call "a death warrant." Czech established she was indeed admitted in July 1941 and killed there in September. "Pneumonia" was the listed cause of death.

Hamburger published a book in 1939 on the neuroses of childhood.[124] In it he elaborated at great length on childhood mental illness with over twenty case studies in a chapter called "Neuroses of the Central Nervous System." Little Professors are nowhere to be found here; simply epilepsy, aggressiveness, and phobias. Hamburger seemed quite taken with the benefits of phenobarbital as a treatment, so the notion that the same drug would be used to euthanize "defective" children is clearly plausible.

All this undercuts Silberman's effort to elevate Asperger and the Vienna clinic into larger than life heroes to Kanner's detriment. Silberman paints a gauzy picture—not only had Asperger seen these cases well before anyone else, he protected them, taught them, and was working to discover their unfulfilled potential. To us, unraveling Asperger's motivations seem just about impossible. More importantly, it's not required for our purposes. What remains beyond dispute is the importance of the diagnosis of "autistic psychopathy." The first child Asperger cited in his 1938 speech would be on the borderline of a diagnosis of autism today. If so, this would give Asperger priority in a published document over Kanner.

But there is no sense Kanner was describing intellectually gifted children. He was describing disabled children, most disabled for life, and even those with better outcomes remained severely limited. No wonder there is no evidence Frankl immediately piped up after meeting Donald that they had seen this sort of thing all the time in his own clinic. Clearly, they had not.

◆ ◆ ◆

Deniers use this handful of cases emerging out of the 1920s in Russia and Vienna to argue for autism's ancientness, but we think it shows the opposite. If these cases could be observed and recorded in the medical literature, where was the Kanner kind of autism in which children didn't just make unusual use of language but couldn't speak; who didn't just withdraw to read or be alone but seemed not to recognize other people as humans; and whose perseverations confined them to repetitive thoughts and rituals as tightly as if they were physically shackled?

Something new and ominous was starting to show itself, first in scattered clusters but soon enough in numbers that overran the old diagnoses like Heller's and childhood schizophrenia, creating a new category that today has impacted about 2 percent of all children. This is the plain and simple truth, which requires no speculation, no tendentious collection of facts, and no speculation—no Autism Denial.

◆ ◆ ◆

Silberman quotes Asperger as saying such children were common and some had gone on to productive lives—again, a claim congruent with sparing them from death—and that the clinic had followed some two hundred children over several decades. Yet Asperger, born in 1906, didn't graduate from medical school until 1931 and was not in a position to have followed children for more than a few years by 1944; his case series included only four children; Case 1, Fritz V., was born just three months before Kanner's first patient, Donald T., in June 1938.

Although an Allied bomb destroyed Asperger's records during World War II, there is evidence from subsequent years that Asperger was not seeing a significantly higher number of cases than Kanner. A retrospective analysis[125] of records of "autistic psychopaths" diagnosed by Asperger and his team at the Children's Hospital, Vienna, checked all diagnoses of autism spectrum disorder in every file case in twenty-three boxes archived at the Institute of Medical History. "According to the card file Asperger saw approximately 9,800 children between 1951 and 1980. Two hundred and thirteen children (2.17 percent) had disorders on the autism spectrum."

Yet Silberman paints Kanner as some kind of pharaoh who deigned to see only the most severe cases and hurled the rest into the chasm of the ignored: "In essence, he was sitting at the apex of a pyramid designed to filter all but the most profoundly disabled children of the most well-connected families in America out of his caseload. From this rarefied perspective, it's not surprising that his syndrome seemed both exceptionally rare and strikingly monolithic. The milder cases among the two hundred children seen by Asperger in Vienna would likely have never made it to the top of his pyramid."

But hold on—Kanner and Asperger were both diagnosing about the same number of patients over the years, two hundred or so for Asperger (and that number may be seriously inflated) versus Kanner's one hundred and fifty; the only conclusion can be that the ones Kanner saw were simply more disabled, not by design, but by nature. This is contrary to the idea that Kanner was keeping a horde of less severe cases at bay, the better to claim a novel and severe new disorder as his own discovery. And it's interesting that among those nearly ten thousand children with potential mental disorders that Asperger saw over those many years, just over 2 percent got an autism diagnosis. That's close to the current rate of 1.47 percent of *all* children, suggesting just how uncommon any form of autism was before the explosion that began in the late 1980s and the 1990s. It's hard to argue that Asperger himself was unable to diagnose cases of Asperger's disorder! And why didn't Asperger appear to see any significant number of the severely disabled cases Kanner did? For the same reason van Krevelen fruitlessly kept watch for nearly a decade—they were rare, until they weren't.

Donvan and Zucker, as well as Silberman, spent a lot of time and effort attacking or lionizing Kanner and Asperger. To be sure, neither Kanner nor Asperger were perfect. They were flawed and prey to the worst instincts of their era—following Freud in blaming parents for a child's autism (Kanner) or going along (for whatever mix of motivations) with Nazi overlords (Asperger). We don't see why any of this makes a great deal of difference in the history of autism. Kanner and Asperger happened to be in the right place at the right time—pioneers who linked pediatrics and psychology, at clinics to which concerned observers would refer the most perplexing and difficult cases; they were thus able to make and disseminate a discovery about a new form of mental illness in children. Yet their discoveries were authentic, their case histories carefully recorded, and their colleagues—at first dubious—ultimately corroborated their observations. There is no need to characterize these contributions as either heroic or villainous. The children and the families are in all respects more important than the first qualified observers who described them, none more than Case 1, Donald T.

There are many similarities between the observations of Kanner and Asperger, but also critical differences. In Silberman's effort to demonize Kanner and assign priority to Asperger, we take Kanner's side. Kanner was the first to describe a syndrome. No one saw it before and we've confirmed that. He chose the name emphasizing age of onset and the term autism as a noun. The syndrome was accepted quickly and has not been questioned since.

As for the debate between Silberman, who sees Asperger as his hero, and Donvan and Zucker, who see him as a murderer, we think Donvan and Zucker have the better evidence. Even more to the point, we think Asperger's claim to priority in discovering a novel syndrome is withering as more historical evidence accumulates. Asperger named a syndrome that was observed before; it was merely his name for it that caught on. He happened to use the same word as Kanner but as an adjective in the context of psychopathy, which placed the syndrome in the context of a different class of children. He clearly has less claim to priority in the rights to discovering Little Professors than Sukhareva and Weiss. And while Kanner's syndrome has stood the test of time, Asperger's syndrome was controversial from the start (was eccentricity really a disability worth addressing?) and when accepted, it was clearly differentiated from autism. Now it's no longer accepted in its original form.

As we'll see in the next chapter, the obsession with Asperger's syndrome, carrying with it as it does the hope for a larger and higher-functioning proportion of people with autism than history or facts warrant, has seriously skewed the debate and aided the idea that there's no epidemic, just a "lost tribe" coming into its own.

CHAPTER 5

Unqualified Observers

"Bullshitting is not exactly lying, and bullshit remains bullshit whether it's true or false. The difference lies in the bullshitter's complete disregard for whether what he's saying corresponds to facts in the physical world: he does not reject the authority of the truth, as the liar does, and oppose himself to it. He pays no attention to it at all. By virtue of this, bullshit is a greater enemy of the truth than lies are."

—Harry Frankfurt, Professor of Philosophy, Princeton University, *On Bullshit*

◆ ◆ ◆

Every journalist who has been at it for a while (in Dan's case, four decades or so) has a treasure trove of boneheaded errors they can recount. Mistakes happen. The trick for journalists is to learn how easy it is to get things wrong before we look like complete idiots when it really matters.

By that standard, Steve Silberman, John Donvan, and Caren Zucker look foolish in things that really do matter. Beyond errors in their arguments, they make mistakes in their books that suggest they don't really know what they're talking about.

Donvan and Zucker make fewer mistakes but some that are quite crucial to the "branding" that is so important to them. Silberman's argument is more powerful (which is not especially hard because Donvan and Zucker don't really have one), but his mistakes are more egregious. Some specific mistakes they make invalidate central pieces of their case. Examples? Donvan and Zucker attempt to co-opt their discovery of Donald T. and misrepresent their own claim to journalistic priority in the discovery of "Autism's First Child." And as we've seen, Silberman makes Leo Kanner his central villain and random mad scientists his heroes, but makes jaw-dropping errors and scatters wild speculation in his quest for the perfect narrative.

Why does all this matter? To be sure, some of these mistakes have more to do with the idiosyncratic positions staked out by these three writers than with the true history and prospect of individuals and families touched by autism. But they do speak to the credibility of their arguments. In Silberman's case, a false narrative about "Asperger's lost tribe" is largely based in invalid evidence, so our demonstrating that matters: as the legal dictum goes, "falsus in uno, falsus in omnibus" ("false in one thing, false in everything"). Too much of what Silberman has written is just plain wrong. As for Donvan and Zucker, their quest to tell the definitive "story of autism" deserves opprobrium because so much of what they write is elliptical, overwrought, and self-serving. And like the eminent philosopher Harry Frankfurt, we need to call bullshit on that.

The Importance of Finding Donald T.

In 2005, we identified Donald T. as Donald Gray Triplett of Forest, Mississippi. The tip-off was a short paper by Leo Kanner from the 1970s.[126] He referred to Donald as a bank teller in the small town of Forest, Mississippi—a classic case of too much information in this modern Internet age about a supposedly anonymous medical case study. Looking online for Donald T* in the white pages for Forest, we saw one name and one name only—Donald Triplett, phone and street address given.

A child as disabled as Donald T.—the index case of a striking new condition—now had a house and a listed phone number? We dialed it and got a recording of a perfectly pleasant-sounding older man. After cross-checking other information about his family, we realized this had to be Case 1, Donald T.

After discussing how to approach this discovery, Dan got on a plane and flew to Jackson, then drove into the small town of Forest. We knew that Donald had an older brother, Oliver Beaman Triplett III—known as O.B. (their father went by Beaman). Like his father, O.B. had a law firm on the second floor of a building on the town square. Dan walked in, identified himself, and proceeded to have a conversation we have recounted elsewhere—about how Donald had been severely autistic, but then, in early adolescence, developed a near-fatal case of juvenile rheumatoid arthritis. The treatment—injected gold salts given over a period of months at the famed Campbell Clinic in Memphis—cleared up not just the arthritis but the most severe autism symptoms, allowing Donald to go to college, work at the family's Bank of Forest, and, now in retirement, travel worldwide. In fact, he was out of town during Dan's visit.

"It's the most amazing thing I've ever seen," O.B. told us, attributing the improvement to the gold salts regimen. Dan asked him more than once if the treatment, rather the time he had spent with a kindly farm family when he was taken ill, had made the difference. "It sure did," O.B. said. "He became more social. . . . He just had a miraculous response to the medicine. The pain in his joints went away." Donald has one fused knuckle to show for the nearly fatal affliction.

There was more good news.

"When he was finally released, the nervous condition he was formerly afflicted with was gone," his brother said. "The proclivity to excitability and extreme nervousness had all but cleared up, and after that he went to school and had one more little flare-up (of arthritis) when in junior college."

Then a correspondent for United Press International, Dan wrote up the discovery. The article appeared on August 15, 2005: "The Age of Autism: Case 1 Revisited,"[127] read the headline. "The first person ever diagnosed with autism lived in a small town in Mississippi," the article began. "He still does."

We weren't the only ones to comment on Donald's improvement after his gold salts therapy. John Hopkins has kept in touch with the Tripletts for years, and in 1956, Leon Eisenberg, Kanner's colleague at Hopkins wrote, "On the basis of a tentative diagnosis of Still's disease [JRA], he was placed empirically on gold therapy with marked improvement. . . . The clinical improvement in his behavior . . . was accelerated during and after his illness and convalescence at home."[128]

Dan's article continued: "Donald T is now 71, and after a 'miraculous response' to medical treatment at age 12, he appears to have recovered significantly since his original diagnosis as a 5-year-old."

Dan didn't name him. A few years later, we both visited him in Forest for an in-depth interview that we published in our book, *The Age of Autism*. This time we did name him, using our recorded interview verbatim in our book, whose publication date was September 15, 2010.

We were not, it turned out, the first to interview Donald. A French documentary filmmaker name Anne Georget filmed him a few years earlier and showed him enjoying his favorite avocation, golf.[129] The documentary had Leo Kanner referencing Donald in a speech as a bank teller, but bleeped the mention of Forest. Georget doesn't recall how she got in touch with Donald but said it wasn't through an investigative effort but rather a chance connection with a mother of an autistic child who knew of him. Like our initial reporting, she didn't disclose Donald's last name or hometown in order to protect his privacy.

Two years after we located and wrote about Donald T., John Donvan and Caren Zucker of ABC decided to find him, too. They described the hunt in several interviews. "He shows up in the literature as just Donald T., the name not spelled out, and we decided to find him," Donvan said in an interview on WTTW in Chicago in 2016. "That's where our investigative reporter Caren Zucker comes in because she found him."[130]

"I should tell you how we found Donald," Zucker said.[131] They knew he lived in Forest. "In researching, all we knew was his name was Donald T.—no Triplett, so we decided that I would call all the T's in Forest, Mississippi, and as I got down the list—it wasn't that bad, about a dozen or so—I get an answering machine." The voice ended by saying "Hello! Happy spring!" She knew instinctively this was Donald Triplett, she said.

In a 2010 video for the *Atlantic* magazine, the story John Donvan described was different.[132] "We had kind of heard through the autism grapevine"—mind you, this was two years after Dan's wire service story describing Donald as very much alive—"that maybe Donald was still around. Donald being the boy described by Kanner as Case Number 1. Kanner was a little bit loose with the confidentiality. We knew his birthdate and we knew his first name was Donald and we knew his last name began with a T and we knew he lived in Forest, Mississippi, and we found out that in Forest, Mississippi, a family whose name began with a T had made a contribution to an autism society. And we looked up what was that full name and we went to the phone book and we knew the last name was Triplett, were there any Donald Tripletts, and bingo! There was."

This left us a bit confused. We reached out to Zucker and Donvan for clarification. A month later, Donvan responded: "Caren and I were able to connect last night to discuss. We concur that, given your website's pattern of overt slurs aimed our way, which suggest malice, we'd need to see the full draft chapter before even consider [sic] engaging."[133]

So what really happened? Did the ABC News team find Donald through a check of charity records that led to his hometown, the family name, and thence—bingo!—to "Donald Triplett" in the phone book? Or did they find out somehow that he lived in Forest, Mississippi, and went to the phone book looking for a Donald in the T's.? Given that their public stories don't match, are they concealing some other route to their discovery path?

◆ ◆ ◆

The day before our book featuring Donald came out in 2010, the pair were everywhere with their Donald T. revelation. It was a media/marketing onslaught from the *Atlantic*, NPR, and ABC News, casting the story in "it takes a village" mode. The citizens of Forest, you see, along with Donald's parents, helped Donald become a happy, independent, well-adjusted, beloved member of the community. If only other communities would do the same, people with autism could live happily ever after in a nurturing, accepting world warmed by the golden fire of love.

Zucker: "Donald had a very good life. He grew up in a community, a small community . . . He had the support of a community and community is huge in terms of people with autism being able to be as independent as possible."[134]

On a *Nightline* segment, the anchor shows Donald at his brother's law office and says his journey mirrors that of autism today—"from despair to hope."[135] (This would be news for many families fighting for services or a modicum of understanding when a child has a meltdown in aisle seven or ages out of public education at twenty-two).

In another showcase[136] for their book, ABC's *Good Morning America* anchor George Stephanopoulos showed clips from the heartwarming stories the pair had done since 2001, then said: "You first did this special back in about 2001, and there were about one in every five hundred kids diagnosed with autism. Now it's one in forty-five. Does this mean there is an epidemic?"

"It's not really actually clear that there's an epidemic," Donvan replied. "The truth is that we don't know because we're always comparing apples and oranges. The definition has changed so much. And where we come out on the science on this is we don't know if there is an epidemic. We don't know if there's not an epidemic but we also think that it shouldn't matter when we decide whether to respond to the needs of people in the autism community."

This is pure bullshit in the Frankfurt sense. Who cares what's true? Everyone should just be nice to each other from now on.

"What we should do is really try to focus on the fact that they need respect, they need support, they need us to be inclusive of them." After debunking the "bad science" of a vaccine link to autism, they turn to Donald T., who Zucker called "an example of how good a life can be having autism if your community embraces you."[137]

This pabulum omitted discussion of Donald's biomedical situation—the gold salts treatment as a factor in his improvement. In their book they give it a dismissive footnote in which they misspelled Dan's last name. They suggested that according to Donald's brother O.B., their long-deceased mother believed the fevers brought on by the juvenile rheumatoid arthritis, rather than the treatment for the autoimmune condition itself, aided this permanent, lifelong improvement.[138] The fact that thousands of subsequent parents have reported that biomedical interventions helped their child, and few credit kindly kinfolk and communities with significant, cinematic-style breakthroughs, does not deter the happy tale. Many parents have remarked that fevers do seem to help autistic children's behavior, but the effect lasts only as long as the fever.

Nor do Donvan and Zucker express any interest in why Donald, the central character in the book, was the first case of a disorder they profess not to know or care is an epidemic; where the other sixty autistic people—not just children—in his small hometown might have been hiding themselves in the 1930s; or any other aspect of the rising numbers Stephanopoulos cited.

Admittedly, their focus was on parents fighting to get the best possible treatment and care for their children, and Donald's mother made an inspiring story, though one that has not curbed the suffering of the millions of children worldwide who have followed.

In a taped *Nightline* segment,[139] the anchor introduces Donvan and Zucker's account of Donald, including his mother's efforts to get him diagnosed at the leading psychiatric hospital in the country. That was a bold and loving act. But this is wishful schmaltz: "It's the diagnosis that changed one person's life and the course of medical history, the first diagnosed case of autism—a life forever changed and one mother whose journey helped millions of families and children who followed."

So millions of families and children followed autism's Case 1 over the course of seventy-five years, but we don't know or care if this is an epidemic? Donvan and Zucker can't have it both ways: if there's no epidemic, then there's nothing special about Donald T. and the entire arc of their lengthy book, which begins and ends with Donald, is deranged; if there is an epidemic, then their appropriation of Donald's story for a "Person of the Week" feature trivializes his importance and betrays the community of parents they purport to celebrate. In our view, Donald's real importance, as well as the importance of the other ten families in Kanner's original case series, lies not in the lessons of love that surrounded him but rather in the clues his environment provides to the cause of the autism crisis. Donvan and Zucker want to make people cry and give money to help families with autism; real help will only come from acknowledging and ending the epidemic, based on clear-cut evidence of its reality, its recency, its severity, and its environmental origins. Donald is crucial for that understanding, but in Donvan and Zucker's treacly narrative, he stands exploited.

Careless Insinuations

If Donvan and Zucker are guilty of distorting the importance and narrative around Donald Triplett, they are at least correct on most of their facts. By contrast, Silberman, whose argument is a more straightforward and unabashed form of Epidemic Denial, often gets the facts wrong when he's not concocting fabulous speculations that rely on no evidence whatsoever. Two examples are worth mentioning: one in Kanner's history and one in another central figure in *NeuroTribes*.

It is difficult to understand, yet alone support, Silberman's antipathy for Kanner. Yes, he was flawed, and speculating as he did that "refrigerator" parents played a major role in creating their child's autism was inexcusable. But to turn that into a narrative in which he skewed the history of autism by effectively burying the less severely affected cases is quite another category of culpability.

To show how far Silberman goes, let's look at an episode we are familiar with from our book *The Age of Autism*. The way Silberman tells the story is completely garbled and in the most critical respects just plain wrong. We reported[140] that Kanner migrated to the United States in 1925 to pursue his career in psychiatry. He landed at the Yankton State Hospital in the middle of nowhere for an ambitious psychiatrist, but he immediately set about using his keen observational skills to write medical journal papers and, no doubt, make a name for himself (not a crime in any of the fifty states) and get straight out of Yankton.

To make a short story of it, Silberman completely confuses the way Kanner went about looking for a neurological form of syphilis in Native Americans. The facts: the famed Emil Kraepelin, who we described in chapter 1, came to Yankton as part of a worldwide study of Indians with general paresis of the insane, known as GPI. That's a late stage, fatal, god-awful form of syphilis. No one knew what caused it to occur in a small percentage of those already infected with syphilis years before, but Kraepelin thought it was alcohol—and Kraepelin wrote in 1913 that it was remarkable "with what extraordinary rapidity paresis has spread among the . . . Indians of North America."

The stage was quite clearly set: Kraepelin thought alcohol caused GPI, and that Indians had an alcohol problem, and that there was a lot of GPI on Indian reservations.

But on a trip to the Americas he was finding none. There did happen to be one Native American with GPI at Kanner's Yankton hospital—a fully Americanized Native American, Thomas Robertson. That struck Kanner as notable—just one Indian, not a ward full suffering from GPI if Kraepelin was correct.

Kanner, aware of Kraepelin's impending visit, took the initiative to look at published papers and contact a wide range of qualified observers, including the surgeon general of the United States, looking for instances of GPI in Native Americans. He found no other cases, and when he met Kraepelin, he told him so. The great psychiatrist was impressed with the upstart and told him he should publish his findings.

Not bad for a twenty-five-year-old psychiatrist who just two years earlier had been a cardiologist living in Berlin. But Silberman tries to make this an early example of Kanner overdramatizing his findings, calling attention to himself and getting things just plain wrong:

"Kraepelin and Plaut [his assistant] were convinced that paresis was extremely rare among blacks and Native Americans, despite the fact that rates of syphilis infection in these groups were high.[141]

Wrong. They did not think paresis (GPI) was rare among blacks or Indians. They thought it was common. Kanner showed that simply wasn't true. *It was uncommon.* But Silberman plunged confidently in the wrong direction, dragging Kanner's reputation behind him.

"The following year, Kanner and Adams published a paper in the *American Journal of Psychiatry* based on their study of this allegedly unusual patient [Thomas Robertson]. The authorial voice is unmistakably Kanner's. He reports that the incidence of paresis is so low among Native Americans that not a single case has 'been heretofore reported in literature,' a phrase he would echo nearly verbatim in his first paper on autism. In fact, he declares, 'such a case is so rare, that it is really regarded as a curiosity, a fact that very decidedly calls for explanation.'" Silberman also digs up a counterargument to Kanner's observation, which simply makes the former look tendentious and the latter look like an earnest researcher using the best evidence available at the time.

Here Silberman sets up Kanner as a factually impaired blowhard with "a flair for dramatic narrative" that we are meant to believe will inform and skew his far-more important work on autism in just a few years. And he fails to grasp Kanner's point that a single instance or a few scattered cases of a disorder is often not evidence of its ubiquity but rather its novelty (the "bearded-lady effect"). The same point applies with equal force when the first few autism and Asperger's cases surfaced, and the same misunderstanding leads Silberman to miss the fact that it heralded an incipient epidemic, rather than demonstrating a steady-state disorder.

Get something wrong and then use it to whale on the person who got it right and everything that person has done ever since? Not good. Silberman demonstrates his characteristic carelessness here. His sole citation for this episode refers to a report from Kraepelin's colleague that was written after the visit, and after Kanner's publication. It reflected on the lessons from their trip, not the reasons they embarked on it, stating once again as plain as day that they found that "general paralysis is also decidedly rare among the North American Indians."

◆ ◆ ◆

Silberman's own forays into the prehistory of Asperger's[142] are not much more rewarding. *NeuroTribes'* chapter one, "The Wizard of Clapham Commons," opens with an eleven-page portrait of Henry Cavendish, a British scientist born in 1731 who discovered hydrogen, developed the thermometer, and helped pioneer the scientific method. Silberman speculates (as ever) that he was an early case of Asperger's disorder, relying for this ersatz diagnosis on contemporary accounts that painted him as eccentric and pathologically shy.

"Cavendish was a great man, but with extraordinary singularities," wrote Henry Lawson, a friend. "His voice was squeaking, his manner nervous, he was afraid of strangers and seemed, when embarrassed, even to articulate with difficulty. He wore the costume of our grandfathers; was enormously rich, but made no use of his wealth. . . . He lived latterly the life of a solitary."[143] And so on.

Ergo, he must have had Asperger's, a suggestion first made by the late psychiatrist Oliver Sacks, who also provides the introduction for Silberman's book. Yet all we know of Cavendish's early years, from his first biographer George Wilson, is that he attended Cambridge but didn't graduate—nothing about whether he had any of the symptoms of Asperger's at the requisite early age. He then returned to London to live with his wealthy father, Charles, where he set up his first chemistry lab in the house. After his father died, he moved into another home where he built an even more elaborate lab.

An elaborate chemistry lab in a private home presided over by a college dropout? Today, that sentence would be followed by an evacuation order. Yet Cavendish merrily brewed up endless experiments involving toxic metals such as arsenic and mercury. In 1783, he wrote a paper titled "Observations on Mr. Hutchins's Experiments for Determining the Degree of Cold at Which Quicksilver Freezes" on the properties of elemental mercury;[144] the word mercury appears forty-five times in Wilson's biography (quicksilver, a synonym, appears nineteen times).[145]

In 1805, the same era as Cavendish's mad metals mixing, John Pearson described a disorder he named erethism, the principal manifestations of which were "excessive timidity, diffidence, increasing shyness, loss of self-confidence, anxiety, and a desire to remain unobserved and unobtrusive. The victim also had a pathological fear of ridicule and oft reacted with an explosive temper when criticized."[146] That sure sounds like Cavendish. Erethism is caused by exposure to mercury vapor. If you wanted to make a case for mercury-induced erethism in a seventeenth-century scientist, Cavendish would be your man. Instead, Silberman has chosen him as Exhibit A in his case that Asperger's has always been around and autism is not an epidemic. He never mentions Cavendish's lifetime of exposure to toxic metals.

We won't speculate on what made Cavendish act the way he did. Silberman will—and gladly.

Neuro-nonsense

Both books are notably weak on the simple facts that surround the debate over the role vaccination may have played in the rise in autism. This debate is not the purpose of our argument here, but the same legal dictum, "falsus in uno, falsus in omnibus," applies to their similarly dismissive arguments. They both regard the vaccine-autism link as unscientific drivel aided by unscrupulous doctors—most often, the uniquely evil Andrew Wakefield—unworthy, apparently, of mastering the argument in any depth.

In *NeuroTribes*, Silberman says that parents were the first to raise concern about mercury in vaccines. Wrong—it was the government.

Silberman: "After an outcry from organizations like (Barbara Loe) Fisher's National Vaccine Information Center, the Centers for Disease Control in Atlanta and the American Academy of Pediatrics asked vaccine manufacturers to remove thimerosal from their products. . . . "[147]

No, no, no! In 1997, the FDA was ordered by Congress to look at medicines that contained mercury. The FDA analysis of the unintentional excessive levels of the ethyl mercury preservative thimerosal in vaccines led in turn to the Public Health Service announcement in 1999 that phased out thimerosal's use in childhood vaccines (they're still in flu shots).[148] Only then was there a (quite justifiable) outcry from parents. Parents were the first to make public the link to autism, but the CDC was already investigating the connection and (only in private) finding it quite plausible.

You make this kind of mistake when you think the idea that mercury might be dangerous in vaccines is so absurd that the crazy anti-vaccine parents must have started it and when you think Fisher is a wild-eyed loon whose lunacy can help you make whatever opposite point you want: the idea, for example, that the original CDC investigator found the thimerosal link to autism not only plausible but likely ("Personally, I have three hypotheses," said CDC analyst Thomas Verstraeten in a secret June 2000 meeting. "Third hypothesis? It's true. It's thimerosal."[149]) is a detail Silberman considers beneath mentioning.

Ditto *In a Different Key*. The authors report that in response to 9/11, Congress added the infamous "Eli Lilly rider" to the bill creating the Department of Homeland Security, sparing Eli Lilly from liability for its use of thimerosal in vaccines.

"The discovery of the rider caused a brief outcry," they write. "Families were now obliged to pursue their cases through a process known as vaccine court."[150]

Again, no. Donovan and Zucker appear not to know that the "Lilly rider" was repealed under massive public pressure in response to its blatant special-interest overreach (protecting Eli Lilly), and not just from anti-vaccine nut jobs but by majorities of both houses of Congress.[151] Thus, it had no effect on whether families were obliged to pursue their cases through vaccine court. (That was the result of a law passed in 1986.)

In a Different Key also mangles the other foundational issue for vaccine safety concerns—Dr. Andrew Wakefield's *Lancet* study in 1998. According to Zucker and Donvan, the study reported that, "the measles virus was present in all 12 children."[152]

Wrong again! If you're going to spend seven years on this book and make a dismissal of the vaccine hypothesis championed by thousands of parents one of your central purposes (they devote over fifty pages to the task), read the damn paper! We sent their passage to Wakefield, who commented, correctly: "Absolute garbage! The *Lancet* paper makes no reference to detection of measles virus. A later paper by Kawashima from Japan, on blinded samples of cases and controls, found measles genetic material in some autistic children. He published this result."[153]

But of course, since Wakefield is a fraud and since the only issue is that solitary paper (Wakefield and colleagues published numerous related papers; dozens of papers provide supportive evidence), he must have said that in that one infamous paper! In the same key, because there is no autism epidemic, all data must be read and presented in such a way as to undercut it. History is built of blocks called facts. Before you try to interpret the edifice they create, you need to make sure the foundation is solid.

Given these goofs, how much should we rely on the depth of their understanding of the autism-as-epidemic argument? How much should we care about Donvan and Zucker's column in the *Washington Post* last year doling out tips to presidential candidates and calling a vaccine link "scaremongering"?[154]

"The autism world, like the world in general, needs less discord," they write, in the kumbaya style that suits their mistake-prone view of autism's history. No! The autism world needs a loud and persistent revolution with as much unpleasantness as is required (in Rimland's words) to find the truth and help sick kids.

Van Krevelen's Revelation

Though you'd never know it, given the starkly different emphases of the two books, the worlds of Kanner's autism and Asperger's disorder began to be understood in context decades ago. First there had to be enough of each to actually tease out both the similarity in kind and the difference in severity.

One further error both books make returns us to the central issue of denying the epidemic. There was clearly a recognition of autism as it arrived; both "full-syndrome," or Kanner autism as it was initially called, as well as Asperger's Little Professors were new and, in Kanner's memorable phrase, "markedly and uniquely different from anything reported so far." But many questions remained wrapped inside those categories, including whether they had been seen before (Little Professors, yes; Kanner autism, no), and how they were different from each other. Were they parts of the same disorder or not? What to make of all the cases of affected children who didn't quite match Kanner's strict profile?

For a long time, children who didn't fall neatly into either category—not Little Professors but not the most severe cases, either—were often called atypical autism; there were many early studies of affected but less severe children.

Both books respond to this widening presentation of severe autism traits by celebrating the hypothesis that there was a spectrum of autism, most famously put forward by Lorna Wing in 1981. In the process, they leave out a whole different side of the debate in the community, one that we see as far more important because it dealt with the sharp profiles of Asperger's and autism when the numbers were low and the differences between Little Professors, who were often prodigies, and disabled children who never spoke, were striking.

In 1952, Arn van Krevelan in Holland saw his first case of autism.

"It took nearly nine years before the first case of 'early infantile autism' was published in Europe," van Krevelen later wrote.[155] "Being well aware of Kanner's publications, I was able to arrive at the diagnosis when I happened upon the parents of an autistic child. I noticed at the time that one could hardly ask for more accurate informants than the parents of an autistic child." In a letter to Rimland, he wrote, each child was "as much like those described by Kanner as one raindrop is like another."[156]

Van Krevelen was not alone in his skepticism while he waited to see evidence of this supposed new disorder, further signs of its rarity in the early period after it was first reported. When Leo Kanner published his case series in April 1943, he quickly had to contend with that era's version of Epidemic Denial, questioning the validity of autism as a differential diagnosis from childhood schizophrenia.

Louise Despert, who we introduced in the last chapter, wrote to say "I object to the coining of new terminology for entities which, while perhaps not so carefully described, have been previously reported. Grebelskaya-Albatz, Ssucharewa, Lutz and even I have reported on early childhood schizophrenia with insidious onset, the symptomatology of which is in all respects similar to the entity you describe."[157] In less formal terms, she's telling Kanner, "You ain't got nuthin."

Kanner wrote back that he did indeed have something. "I have, as is inevitable, seen typical schizophrenic children at a very early age. . . . I fully agree with you that no age limit should or can be set for the onset of schizophrenic withdrawal." Then he played his ace. "At the same time, what strikes me in the group which I have discussed in my paper is the apparent disability from the beginning of life to form adequate affective contact rather than withdrawal from adequate or near-adequate contact already established. This is essentially the thing which, in my mind, sets this group off from other infantile schizophrenics of my acquaintance or those reported in the literature."[158]

In his November 1944 letter to Despert,[159] he was sounding even more confident: "The whole picture no doubt bears resemblance to what is usually combined under the heading of schizophrenia. At the same time, I have come more and more to feel that regardless of classification or nomenclature, these children deserve to be viewed as a more or less specific group." That same year, he came up with the phrase "early infantile autism." By then he had "collected 23 children [double the original case series] who undoubtedly belong to this group." Remember, that's almost the same number—twenty-eight—that Heller had collected of the disorder named for him in twenty-three years.

The correspondence between Despert and Kanner reflects a dialogue that was going on throughout the field of child psychiatry beginning in the 1940s. As Kanner and Asperger were leading the way in describing "markedly and uniquely different" conditions, other qualified observers were seeing similar childhood populations and struggling to make sense of what they were observing. It's one thing to describe (or distort) the history of the discoverers; it's quite another to describe the transformation of the field and the community of practice. In the case of autism, its novelty required adaptation from the community of caregivers.

But as autism cases began to present themselves to qualified observers, the leading practitioners adapted quickly. New York City was one such community where we can observe a rapid change in diagnostic practices. As late as 1933, Howard Potter published an article[160] on schizophrenia in children (citing six cases with age of onset between three-and-a-half and nine years old. Within a few years Despert, also in New York, was debating Kanner about whether his observation was new and eventually conceded she didn't see symptoms that early. By 1947, Lauretta Bender was developing a systematic parsing of New York children, distinguishing clearly between Potter's childhood schizophrenics, Heller's *dementia infantilis*, and Kanner's "autistic disturbances of affective contact," which she actually quoted.

In London, R. A. Q. Lay wrote his 1938 review paper, diving deeply into *dementia infantilis* and childhood schizophrenia. There was no mention of autism. A year earlier, Mildred Creak was also writing from London of "Psychoses in Children."[161] Nothing resembled autism and her definition of childhood onset was even later than Lay's.

Across the channel, as we've seen, much of the pioneering work on child mental disorders was carried out in Germany and Austria. Jacob Lutz thought childhood schizophrenia was rare; August Homburger—another Viennese psychiatrist, but not Asperger's mentor Hamburger—wrote a textbook on child psychiatric conditions and mentions only Heller and Weygandt.

Further east, in Moscow, the situation was not much different. E. Grebelskaja-Albatz reported in 1934 and 1935 on numerous cases of *dementia infantilis*, with a sprinkling of later-onset cases that were more likely childhood schizophrenia.[162] She reported on nothing like autism. The interesting anomaly in Moscow was Sukhareva, who was the first anywhere in the world to report on her Little Professors—"personality disorder: schizoid; (eccentric)" in 1926.

Two decades later, Asperger described three or four such cases while Sukhareva's case series made barely a ripple. Asperger, perhaps because he used the term autistic—the same term Kanner used—gained greater notoriety for his report. Interestingly, it wasn't until much later, with

Franklin Robinson and Louis Vitale writing in 1954,[163] that we see an American report of Little Professors. Was this because the condition was less prevalent or because the Little Professors were so close to normal it didn't seem worth the effort to describe them?

An American report came from Wyoming Valley in Wilkes-Barre, Pennsylvania, and was aptly titled "Children with Circumscribed Interests."

The cases described by the authors were dead ringers for the kind of children Sukhareva, Asperger, and others had begun identifying: "They develop special interests and sometimes special abilities. Their interests are restricted to certain classes of information of types of activity which have special value for the patient. These interests are pursued with a concomitant withholding of interest or endeavor in other types of activity or areas of thought. There is a restriction of social interest and a limited establishment of interpersonal relationships."

Three children were described: the oldest, Tom, was thirteen, so born around 1940. Typically, his problems weren't recognized until age five and kindergarten. "He remained by himself and was unable to participate in activities with other children. In school his social withdrawal continued." He learned to read quickly and became fascinated with chemistry. Other children began to shun him.

And so it went for the three cases studies. (These, by the way, are what real case histories feel like—a clear sense of onset, relationships, and development, not the glancing references that Epidemic Deniers use to claim autism was spotted far and wide before 1930.)

In summary, the authors note "these children call to mind the syndrome described by Kanner under the designation of 'Early Infantile Autism.' They are distinguished from autistic children in that they have not presented the early infantile incapacity of emotional responsiveness. The parents have considered them to have been 'normal babies.' Their interests are circumscribed but their ability to react emotionally is not deficient. They present a lesser degree of 'withdrawal from contact with people' and a lesser measure of the 'obsessive desire for the preservation of sameness' that is encountered in children who have been autistic from early infancy." They usually come to clinical attention between ages eight and eleven. "They are of average or better intelligence."

Kanner himself leads off the comment section and notes other case histories of similar children, including a group in Israel. He remarks that circumscribed interests are present in much greater intensity in autistic children but otherwise it seems that "the syndrome of circumscribed interest patterns" is treated as a separate syndrome.

Clearly, recognition for the Little Professor profile was rising in the United States while the difference between the two disorders was also emerging.

◆ ◆ ◆

In a 1971 article, "Early Infantile Autism and Autistic,"[164] van Krevelen wrote that "New discoveries are period-bound rather than area-bound; they often emerge at the same time in different geographic sections. The history of autism offers a striking example" (given Kanner's 1943 paper in Baltimore and Asperger's 1944 paper in Vienna). "We can take it for granted that neither was then aware of the others' work."

In 1962, he had outlined two distinguishing features between the groups: "Kanner described psychotic *processes,* characterized by a course ... Asperger's autistic psychopathy represents traits, which were static; the patient has an abnormal personality with less sensitivity,

---

All this makes it unmistakably clear that early infantile autism and autistic psychopathy are two entirely different nosological syndromes. The following schema may help to list the major distinguishing features:

Early infantile autism	Autistic psychopathy
1. Manifestation age: first month of life.	1. Manifestation age: third year of life or later.
2. Child walks earlier than he speaks; speech is retarded or absent.	2. Child walks late, speaks earlier.
3. Language does not attain the function of communication.	3. Language aims at communication but remains "one-way traffic."
4. Eye contact: other people do not exist.	4. Eye contact: other people are evaded.
5. The child lives in a world of his own.	5. The child lives in our world in his own way.
6. Social prognosis is poor.	6. Social prognosis is rather good.
7. A psychotic process.	7. A personality trait.

more rationality. The approach is a merely cerebral one. What he lacks is understanding of, and interaction with, people's feelings."[165]

He notes that Asperger's is often spotted in the first years of school whereas in autism it is always apparent in infancy. "All this makes it unmistakably clear that early infantile autism and autistic psychopathy (Asperger's) are two entirely different nosological syndromes."

He put together an invaluable chart:

In Leo Kanner's archive at the Hopkins Medical School is an undated newspaper article that suggests Kanner was as surprised as anyone when he saw his first Little Professor in person. "Hopkins Doctor Tells of Maryland Boy, 4, Who 'Read' English and German."[166]

"The unusual case of a Maryland boy who 'read' both English and German at the age of four—although he couldn't speak German and didn't know what he [was] reading in English—was discussed in a recent paper by Dr. Leo Kanner, psychiatrist in charge of the children's psychiatric outpatient service at Johns Hopkins Hospital."

Kanner said he was first asked to see the child about eight years before. "In a combined library and music room I found a little boy reading aloud from a magazine written for well-educated adults. He paid no attention to my greeting and it was soon obvious the words he read aloud, and fluently, had no meaning for him." Any interference provoked tantrums.

Kanner described how, over a period of years and working with the family, the boy was redirected from his "idiot savant" destiny and now, at twelve, attended junior high school. "He is still a peculiar child, pre-occupied with mathematical puzzles and the collection of maps, but he has a reasonably good relationship with his mother, his sister and his teachers, and has made a few friends."

We find this account revealing, even though we don't know the date, because Kanner was neither hiding nor hyping his observation of a Little Professor. One would think if he were trying to steer the entire autism field toward the most severe cases and away from anything that would point to a wider spectrum, this article, and the paper it derived from, would never have been written, whatever its date.

In our view, the Little Professors and "Kanner's autism," as it was often called, are related but clearly distinct entities. Little Professors have a different natural history and certainly are more difficult to distinguish from introversion and eccentricity. As we'll see, this became a central point of confusion in the debate over autism's rise. Silberman exploits this ambiguity; Donvan and Zucker declare it unimportant and unknowable, apples and oranges. But that is simply false; as we'll see, it is not that hard to count from effectively zero to one in sixty-eight, applying the same criteria all along the way.

The challenges of Little Professors deserve our sympathy and support; that shouldn't create a cover story to ignore the greatest childhood health crisis of our time. It would take until 1994 for Asperger's to become part of the official autism spectrum, and even then, whenever it was counted alongside the more severe cases, it remained a minority of the total, nowhere near enough to begin to explain the avalanche of cases that occurred in the 1990s, the subject of the next chapter.

6/29/2018

LOPEZ JEANNIE

Item Number: 31901032358113

Hold Shelf Slip

CHAPTER 6

The Epidemic and Its Implications

"There are very few things we're discovering that those guys didn't write about, except autism."
> —*Vaxxed* producer Del Bigtree on the lack of mention of autism in medical reports before 1930.[167]

For someone who has been called "the most powerful psychiatrist in America," Allen Frances wears his *eminence grise* well, dark button-down shirt open at the collar and dark sport coat casually setting off a healthy thatch of white hair. His manner matches: unique among the speakers we'd seen at the Real Truth About Health conference in Orlando in September 2016, he leans informally into the lectern, talks without notes, props, or PowerPoint, distilling a lifetime of experience into a conversational but authoritative style. He seems every bit the author of 2013's "Saving Normal—An insider's revolt against out-of-control psychiatric diagnosis, DSM-5, big pharma, and the medicalization of ordinary life."[168]

Frances positions himself against mainstream medicine's follies and excess. The best way to grow old in good health? Avoid two bad things: falls—the leading cause of accidental death—and doctors, whom he implies are not far behind. He mocks his profession's tendency to overdiagnose, overprescribe and, in general, overdo it, turning ordinary sadness or elevated blood sugar results into pre-this and incipient-that, starting the patient down a path to fully medicated, officially certified ill health. He had the audience of flip-flopped, baseball-hatted, Hawaiian-shirted, alternative health types in Orlando firmly on his side. Finally, a doctor who saw the light.

Until, that is, he casually remarked that autism is just another one of those overdiagnosed disorders. The room tensed up—you could feel a chill as if the air-conditioning dropped five degrees. Many of his listeners view autism as a man-made and largely iatrogenic (medically induced) epidemic. Some in the room had seen it happen. This was personal—theirs were the children of the epidemic Frances was denying.

Dan asked the first question.

"Do you think there's been any real increase—"

"You're going to have to speak up because I have really old ears—"

"OK, do you think there's been any real increase in the rate of autism in recent years—or at all?"

Expansion—or Exaggeration

Before we hear from Frances (the exchange is lightly edited for clarity), let's acknowledge our appreciation for the civil and engaged discussion, which brought the strongest arguments *for* Epidemic Denial into high relief from one of the most knowledgeable sources possible (even though we disagree).

Other than schmaltz (Donvan and Zucker's "it takes a village" for autistic kids to thrive) and speculation (Silberman's "lost tribe" coming out of hiding after Leo Kanner's one-man effort to suppress it), the remaining flavor of Denial is that Science-With-A-Capital-S proves there is no epidemic—it's all just "better diagnosing," as we explained in the introduction. Like ancient Gaul, that argument is divided into three: that we just didn't notice autistic people before 1930; that autism was simply substituted for other disorders, notably mental incapacity; and that broadening the criteria—particularly the inclusion of Asperger's in the psychiatrist's diagnostic bible in 1994 (the DSM-IV)—sent cases soaring. We call this triad of Denial hypotheses diagnostic oversight, diagnostic substitution, and diagnostic expansion, and we'll deal with the modern form of each below, just as we've dealt with them in our search for autism before 1930 in earlier chapters. There is also a white-elephant grab bag of other explanations, from the movie *Rain Man* provoking the epidemic to—we kid you not—a "fateful typo" seeming to send rates soaring. We'll run these to ground as well, though, in the immortal phrase of our *Age of Autism* UK editor John Stone, in many cases they and their purveyors "deserve our bristling contempt."

◆ ◆ ◆

Let's start with the DSM changes in 1994, an exercise that updated the 1987 version of the manual, DSM-III Revised, into the next edition, DSM-IV, which Frances oversaw. Frances was certainly an eminent choice for the job, which involved reviewing every one of ninety-four diagnostic categories for mental disorders, from schizophrenia to substance abuse and from depression to hypomania. An emeritus professor and former chair of the Department of Psychiatry and Behavioral Science at Duke University School of Medicine, he had been on the leadership team for the DSM-III and its revision, the DSM-III-R before being named head of the DSM-IV task force. While the acronyms, Roman numerals, and nomenclature sound esoteric, the resulting text has profound real-world consequences: who gets diagnosed with what mental illness, what special provisions are made for education, the kinds of treatments that are appropriate, and how treatment is compensated (if at all), Society, one might even say, gets a sense of itself from the DSM, as it reports that, for example, 15 percent of Americans suffer from depression every year. So calling Frances the most powerful psychiatrist in America due to his DSM work was no exaggeration. But as might be expected from his talk in Orlando, he wielded that power judiciously, even minimally—allowing changes to just two diagnostic categories: bipolar II and the Pervasive Developmental Disorders (PDD), informally known as the autism spectrum.

The main thing DSM-IV did to the PDDs category was pretty simple to understand—for the first time, Asperger's disorder was included. Period. The end. Asperger's simply joined the umbrella category of Pervasive Developmental Disorders, along with the full-syndrome Autistic Disorder and the slightly less devastating Pervasive Developmental Disorders/Not Otherwise Specified (as well as Heller's disorder, now called Childhood Disintegrative Disorder, and a genetic disorder called Rett's that affects only girls; the latter two by the 1990s made a minuscule portion of the overall caseload). Some called Asperger's "autism lite" because, while it certainly imposed limitations and hardships, it was not categorically disabling as was full-syndrome autism (PDD/Autistic Disorder). Thus, from the beginning, DSM-IV extended the spectrum in a way that, at its further edges, could fray into eccentric behavior or self-diagnosis. But could that explain an exponential increase in autism?

Frances thinks so.

◆ ◆ ◆

"There's no gold standard in psychiatry," Frances began his answer to Dan about whether the rise in cases was real. "There are no tests to make any of these diagnoses. So who knows? What I do know is how easy it is to change the rate of a disorder. I mean, we wrote a new disorder—we set criteria for Asperger's—and boom, the diagno[ses] [go] up. School services are tied to it. Boom, they go up."

In other words, Frances argues, the simple step of adding Asperger's raised up a Mount Kilimanjaro of autism cases out of the arid plain that had previously stretched for miles in every direction. But why? Frances had answers. Lots of them. For one, such a diagnosis made it easier to get special accommodations, specifically in school.

"When I'm speaking about the school services I'm not talking about the infantile severe autistic behavior. What I am talking about is the Asperger kid. And in many jurisdictions—it has been looked at in California very carefully—in many jurisdictions where the rates of autism have gone up, it's not in the severe kids who have the early onset."

Well, no. California tracks the severe kids.

"That's not true," Mark replied. "In the California Department of Developmental Services [DDS], that's among the most restrictive definition of all the states around the country. It's not Asperger's. That's not how kids get into the service system in California. If you're going to make claims like that—that's an aggressive claim—don't do it casually."

Frances: "It is possible we could disagree. There may not be a clear right and wrong in this."

In fact, there is. In terms of the widely circulated one in sixty-eight prevalence number (the current estimate from the CDC's surveillance for the 2002–04 birth years), adding Asperger's expanded the effective diagnostic reach of the DSM-IV by roughly 10 percent—enough for an arithmetic increase proportionate to the category expansion but not an exponential one—ten, twenty, one hundred times—that kept rising every year. That's just the CDC number.[169] The 1999 California study (more on this below) included a category that captured Asperger's syndrome (it went up nearly 2,000 percent), but that wasn't the increase that DDS reported: that increase measured only PDD/Autistic Disorder and was 273 percent (3.7 times) in eleven years.[170] In all respects, when assessing the impact of adding Asperger's, all one has to do is make sure to know whether or not Asperger's cases are added to the numbers one is considering. In most cases, the scary autism numbers we hear aren't affected very much by Asperger's cases. But the Deniers aren't interested in accuracy; they want everyone to be confused rather than deeply concerned.

Frances elaborated on the changes he oversaw.

"Let me explain what we did with DSM-IV—so you understand the thinking. We had a very high standard for making changes in DSM-IV. We didn't want to change the system. . . . We only made two changes with new diagnoses. One was adding Asperger's [to the Pervasive Developmental Disorders category that includes autistic disorder] and the other was adding bipolar 2—two out of ninety-four, we were very selective in making changes."

"Very selective" is right. Frances was not hell-bent on using his power to fiddle with the diagnostic order or leave his stamp on the psychiatric bible. Asperger's addition was not part of some promiscuous expansion of the new manual. The addition of Asperger's syndrome was permitted only because doing so had widespread support. There was clearly something going on with more Little Professors out there in the world, and along with them a rising demand to recognize the milder end of the "autism spectrum." So it was a valid concept that recognized a reality—but also opened the door for a blurring of the harsh world of autistic disorder as it shaded into Asperger's. And it was made to order for Epidemic Deniers who could start talking about apples and oranges and moving the goalposts.

Frances emphasized the change was driven by clinicians and that adding Asperger's was a move to aid frontline doctors in diagnosing patients. But something unexpected happened. Autism rates soared. "There was a very sudden increase, a tremendously sudden increase, in the rates, which used to be between one-in-two thousand and one-in-five thousand. The rates very quickly increased. Before very long it was one in one hundred and twenty, it was one in sixty-eight, there have been some studies in which it was one in thirty-eight."

But why? This is the question at the heart of Epidemic Denial, which Frances proceeded to embrace as he and Mark sparred for the next few minutes.

Frances: "Now either your position might be there was a sudden change that resulted in going from one in two thousand—"

Mark interjected there was indeed such a change, that the spike was real: "Just when you're doing the field trials [for DSM-IV], that was the tipping point, the late 80s."

Frances: "Yes you think there was a sudden change that went from one in two thousand to one in five thousand to one in thirty-eight to one in sixty-eight. . . . "

Mark: "One in thirty-eight is in South Korea, it's not a US number . . . ."

Frances: "And that's the environmental. . . . "

Mark: "Yes. . . . "

Frances: Toxin. . . . "

Well there you have it. Yes, the increase is real, and it reflects an environmental toxin (us). Or, no, it's just broadening the criteria, a subspecies of better diagnosing that allowed in more cases (Frances). It's the critical issue, and it's also a testable hypothesis, and the epidemic wins.

The EPA noted a worldwide spike in autism rates beginning in the 1988–89 birth years; the trend continued and was noticed by the CDC and others just as the new DSM-IV was coming out in 1994, even before the new criteria had been fully absorbed and adopted by clinicians; yet the Deniers' claim is that the DSM did it. *Fail.*

Frances plowed ahead. "On the other hand, the other side of it you should at least hear. The other side of it is that in all my work with psychiatric diagnosis, going back thirty years, what I've seen over and over again, you make the slightest change in the definition, you say it's going to be four criteria or five criteria, you add a criteria, you subtract a criteria, you have a different type of person doing the evaluation, whether it's done in the research clinic with very long evaluations that are done with semi-structured interviews over time, maybe several weeks, versus someone who does it who has a master's degree who is working very quickly under pressure, maybe not so expert, you get tremendous changes in rate with every move you make in the diagnostic system."

◆ ◆ ◆

Yet the history of the DSM-IV provides no basis for the extravagant claim that changes in diagnosis made any substantial difference. In truth, there was nothing special about the 1994 revision of the DSM. First published in 1952, the DSM was revised in 1967 (DSM-II) with no mention of autism. "Infantile autism" was slotted within the broader category of Pervasive Developmental Disorders (PDDs) and first formally included in the third edition, which was published in 1980. Seven years later, the revised third edition was published and with it an update of the DSM criteria for autism (renamed "autistic disorder") and the PDDs. Then, seven years after the revised third edition came the fourth edition, the one Frances oversaw, adding Asperger's as its only material change.

The key point to remember is that the DSM criteria for all "mental disorders" are revised regularly and autism is just one part of this ongoing process. If you read the literature surrounding the autism revisions, you will see that the DSM-IV was never intended to radically expand the definition of autism. Quite the contrary, these revisions are mostly technical publications designed to aid practicing psychiatrists in making consistent diagnoses. But since the timing of this new volume coincided conveniently with the upsurge in autism cases, history has been rewritten. Because as the first children of the Age of Autism were born around 1990 and started receiving their first diagnosis of autism at an average age of four or five, the DSM-IV criteria had, quite naturally, just been introduced.

Yet the overall goal of the designers of the updated autism criteria was in keeping with Frances's strict minimalist philosophy: their goal was not to allow an expansion of the criteria but rather to rein in some of the excesses of the revised third edition in 1987. "Diagnostic systems lose their value if they are either overly broad or overly narrow," wrote Fred Volkmar, a Yale psychiatrist who led the autism revision to the DSM-IV.[171] "They must provide sufficient detail to be used consistently and reliably by clinicians and researchers in varied settings. The change from DSM-III to DSM-III-R is an example of the broadening of the concept of autism; from DSM-III-R to DSM-IV, a corrective narrowing occurred."

Can we all please just pause over this one-sentence counter-narrative to the whole "diagnostic expansion did it" crusade? A corrective narrowing of the criteria for autism occurred. Let's remind ourselves of the criteria in place when Volkmar and crew started working on it in 1994. Michael Rutter's 1978 formulation had built on Leo Kanner's own 1943 observations but systematizing them into the four sides of the fence we described in chapter 3: onset before thirty months; impaired social development; delayed and deviant language development; "insistence on sameness through rituals, abnormal preoccupations, and resistance to change."

Now Asperger's had been added (and the age of onset extended to thirty-six months) and yes, that accounted for more cases. But why did the caseload explode? The reason it exploded and kept going was because that's how many new cases of autism there were, Mark told Frances.

Mark: "The addition of Asperger's was possibly useful and possibly you can find quirky scientific nerdy people, but you don't find what my daughter has, you don't find what thousands and thousands of American people have. In the numbers one in sixty-eight, 10 percent of those kids are Asperger's. Asperger's is a number that has little bearing on these rates."

Frances: Would you say the rest of them are classic childhood autism?"

Mark: "Yes." [Mark misspoke a little here: he should have said the 1 in 68 number included 46 percent PDD/Autistic Disorder and 44 percent PDD/NOS aside from the 10 percent with Asperger's].

Frances: "I think we're going to disagree."

◆ ◆ ◆

The case for updating the criteria after so many years made sense. Not only were more cases being diagnosed by any measure by the 1990s, the variation in cases with what might be described as autistic features and traits had risen significantly. We described how the first American "children with circumscribed interests" were originally described in a published medical paper in 1954; these were Asperger's-type cases, less disabled than the early infantile autism Kanner described but with enough similar features to recognize them as kinfolk. The regressive form—not present in Kanner's first eleven cases (with the possible exception of Case 2, Richard M., who "went backward" at age one around the time of a smallpox vaccination)—surfaced by the 1950s. And children who were clearly disabled by autism but lacked the strict pattern of the defining triad of behavioral symptoms were getting noticed more as well. Thus the ungainly phrase "Pervasive Personality Disorder—Not Otherwise Specified" was adopted, shortened to PDD/NOS.

From Kanner's collection of eleven cases in 1943, why did these variations emerge? In Bernard Rimland's 1964 landmark *Infantile Autism,* in which he showed that parental behavior could not be responsible for autism, one of his arguments for absolving parents was "the absence of blends." In other words, autistic children were so similar—van Krevelen said in 1953 that once he saw them they were as similar as "raindrops" and perfectly fit Kanner's description. If parents caused autism, different degrees of abuse or neglect—different temperatures of "refrigerator parents," as Kanner once called them in his parent-blaming days—should have produced a wider range of cases; instead, autism cases were remarkably similar in severity and symptoms.

So what happened? We believe that with more cases and more exposure to causative substances at different levels and different times, a broader range emerged—the "spectrum" by which autism is now known. The "absence of blends" gave way to a fuller range of behaviors and degrees of disability. These reasonable, rational changes make perfect sense and do not amount, as Deniers say, to "moving the goal-posts." This is what Paul Offit was claiming when we quoted him in the introduction: "It's not an actual epidemic. In the mid-1990s, the definition of autism was broadened to what is now called autism spectrum disorder. People say if you took the current criteria and went back 50 years, you'd see about as many children with autism then."[172]

One is free to believe what one chooses, of course, but on this critical point the evidence is clear. Epidemic Denial fails another test.

Oversight—or Overlooking the Obvious?

As Offit's comment illustrates, the second way Deniers try to claim science is on their side is through "diagnostic oversight"—the idea that autistic people existed (both before and after 1930) but were somehow simply not counted. We believe we've offered quite compelling evidence that the rate of autism before 1930 was effectively zero, but for anything that far back . . . well, many will dismiss evidence that old as just ancient history. Far more relevant is the recent history of autism, after it was discovered and recognized, and the rate of autism in the late twentieth and early twenty-first centuries. To the extent that autism rates were reported in the United States before 1990, the rates were very low: less than one in ten thousand in some cases and never more than one in three thousand. But the Deniers argue that these more recent studies were simply biased and incomplete: the surveys reporting these low rates were primitive and have been rendered obsolete by better surveillance methods. The increasing rates of autism in our lifetime, the Deniers claim, are one of the benefits of progress in scientific methods.

We think that's nonsense. That said, it would be awfully convenient to our own argument if the relevant authorities had spent the time and money to create a more modern survey of the autism rate, one that deployed the gold standard of surveillance methods, a *prospective* study of the autism rate. Such a prospective study would follow a large group of children from birth through childhood, monitoring their development at regular intervals with rigorous consistency to see how they progressed and whether or not they had developmental problems like autism. A prospective study that included autism would tell us what the real autism rate was by carefully tracking a defined population, not by looking back retrospectively trying to identify cases in a population after their onset had already occurred. Ideally, to make a compelling case for low rates of autism before the onset of any purported "epidemic," such a study should have been done somewhere between the recognition of autism in the 1930s and its explosion in the 1990s.

Another ideal feature of such a study would be a large sample size—tens of thousands of children tracked from birth to see what percent were diagnosed with autism. This dream study would cull data from computerized medical records and also from neurological, psychological, speech, and hearing exams at every stage in child development. Top medical centers, leading researchers, and strict government supervision would ensure no conflicts of interest. Compare this mythical study to today's rates and you'd really know if there is an autism epidemic, a mild tick upward, or nothing at all but a change in the gestalt—in the way we describe the varieties of human disability.

Oh, wait. That study *was* done.

It was called the National Collaborative Perinatal Project, the first of its kind. Instead of forcing health researchers to look backwards to assess health outcomes in children, this prospective health assessment project followed a population of newborn babies and rigorously monitored their development along numerous fronts. For an interested researcher, the National Collaborative Perinatal Project allowed the analysis of the computerized records of thirty thousand children—a huge sample—born between 1959 and 1965 at fourteen university-affiliated medical centers. All the children received—at precisely defined intervals—a highly structured set of neurological, psychological, speech, and hearing examinations from birth through eight years of age.

In 1975, a team led by E. Fuller Torrey (a prominent researcher who has written extensively on schizophrenia and the treatment of the mentally ill) took a look at this data that had been assembled a decade before to examine the effect of maternal uterine bleeding during pregnancy on the mental development of the children, including autism.[173]

Torrey and colleagues reported that "from this group 14 were selected as conforming to the syndrome of infantile autism." Remember, "this group" comprised thirty thousand children, far beyond what would be required to find a representative number of children with autism, whatever diagnostic criteria was in place. That translated to a rate of 4.7 autistic children per ten thousand. And that jibed with other studies from that era—including one that found exactly the same 4.7 per ten thousand rate in England.

But for completeness, the study authors added in six children who, while not cases of classic autism, might have received the diagnosis because from the records it was clear they were "disturbed, psychotic like psychotic-like, autistic, or [had] childhood schizophrenia." That gave a combined rate of 6.7 per ten thousand, or one in fifteen hundred; today's one in sixty-eight rate for children born in 2008 is twenty-two times higher. Even if you take 10 percent out of the one in sixty-eight for the subsequent inclusion of Asperger's, today's autism rate is *twenty times higher* than the rate Torrey and colleagues carefully calculated for children born a half century ago.

Come on, Epidemic Deniers! It's not just a fad that led to twenty times the number of carefully diagnosed autism cases between a prospective gold standard study in the 1960s and now. The criteria for finding those cases barely budged. The numbers took off in the late 1980s—even before Frances and his team's 1994 report—in a sharp vertical uptick known as a hockey stick.

Torrey's study offers some of the strongest evidence against the idea that autism grew like Topsy because of some supposed upending of the diagnostic order. And again we see how few places there were for such children to hide—fewer than six psychotic or schizophrenic children to add into the mix out of a sample of thirty thousand.

You may recall Donvan and Zucker claiming an "apples and oranges" problem afflicted the ability to determine whether cases had gone up. Well, here you see apples only and a rate that clearly spells out e-p-i-d-e-m-i-c in any language. Yet the idea that autism has in fact increased is supposedly just a matter of the boundaries we put around the diagnostic box. It's amazing that high profile, otherwise independent-minded people like Allen Frances continue to make that case.

◆ ◆ ◆

Torrey's finding, as with almost every other study on autism, focuses on children. There's a reason for that—since autism was a new disorder that began in infancy, it was first noticed in children. This fact again becomes fodder for Silberman's attack on Kanner: "One thing is certain: if the Wizard of Clapham Common [James Cavendish] had managed to construct a time machine in his backyard, beaming himself directly to the waiting room of child psychiatrist Leo Kanner after his announcement of the discovery of autism in 1943, the brusque, cigar-puffing clinician would have sent him down the hall to another clinic. Adults weren't on Kanner's radar at all until much later. . . . "

We've already described Cavendish and the likelihood that he suffered from mercury-induced erethism, not Asperger's, but the speculation—here become "certain"—that Kanner would refuse to see him because he was an adult is mind-bending. First, Kanner was a *child* psychiatrist, but most importantly Kanner saw only children because, in our view, there were effectively zero autism cases born before 1930. This idea of a hidden horde of autistic adults (Gulliver) again shows its emptiness. If one in sixty-eight adults were walking around with autism, somebody would have noticed. Kanner here gets the blame for discovering its earliest manifestations!

But efforts to find and quantify autistic adults are not confined to Silberman. In 2014, a study in England by Traolach S. Brugha[174] and colleagues concluded that one in one hundred adults had autism—a number that, if sustained, would in fact show a similar prevalence in adults and children and therefore no real increase. They accomplished this feat by going door-to-door and interviewing residents about features that could then be mapped against a possible autism diagnosis—although how a survey of adults living independently could reach anyone other than grown-up Little Professors is anyone's guess.

The flaws with this effort were so numerous it's hard to know where to begin. First, the very nature of the interaction—a door-to-door interview survey—demonstrates they weren't even looking for severe autism cases, which as we've shown constitute about 90 percent of the caseload among children today. You'd find eccentrics and geeks and, yes, perhaps some Asperger's cases. And what would be your point? That some UK residents with an ASD diagnosis from the 1930s onward had reached adulthood?

With all that, they found nineteen cases they believed qualified out of a group of six hundred, and eighteen they had screened out as having a greater chance of being on the spectrum. They then applied an opaque weighting scheme multiplying their sample of nineteen to an estimate of the seventy-two autism cases they thought they might have found and then divided that number by a population of 7,300 they might have surveyed, leading to their conclusion of a one in one hundred autism rate (one that they also calculated—with even greater faux precision— was evenly spread across younger and older adults). Our John Stone at Age of Autism has been tearing this finding apart for months.

"Professor Brugha appears quick to suggest there is no increase in ASDs based on a study of 19 cases—his own—which appears less than robust," Stone has written.[175] In several withering takedowns of the methods and claims of this study, Stone points out, among other weaknesses, that: the authors misrepresented as a standard tool their own made-up screening tool, one which didn't work very well; they applied a diagnostic tool designed for "verbally fluent adults" and suggested it was appropriate for a survey of ASD prevalence; they applied the scoring system of the standard diagnostic tool they followed in nonstandard ways; and when they were all done, they pretended (without foundation) that their entire approach had been well tested and validated . . . by themselves. Despite all these weaknesses, the fact that a survey finding nineteen "verbally fluent" but possibly autistic adults has been trumpeted by many as proof that autism is as common among adults is it is in children.

Against the idea of this hidden horde of autistic adults we'd like to repeat the commonsense test that Kanner's eldest case was born in 1931, and that despite his frequent writing about the condition there is no evidence of any older person ever being referred to him or his associates. We've outlined the handful of potential autism cases before the 1930s, but we believe Kanner's report should have generated a flood of people of all ages. A hidden horde should have spilled out into the open, with rediagnoses and recognition—and not just of children.

Instead, the Epidemic Deniers are knocking on doors and hoping Gulliver will answer and say, "I've been waiting for you for 75 years."

There's another commonsense test to apply, courtesy of Torrey and colleague's prospective study of children born in the 1960s. Take the 1965 population of 194 million and apply the full-syndrome autism rate they came up with of 4.7 per one hundred thousand—that would mean 9,259 Americans of all ages were fully autistic. Compare that total of just below ten thousand to over one million now, most of them still children.

Substitution or Silliness?

The third claim of "better diagnosing" as the explanation for the rise in autism is diagnostic substitution—which we also took up with Frances. Some of the rise, he told us, "is clearly due to the change in diagnostic habits around intellectual disability."

The recognition of autism, and its subsequent increase, was thus a "change in gestalt," or, to put it less loftily, a "fad" in describing a particular kind of human distress. Once again, it seems to us that Epidemic Denial has shown its fundamental emptiness, because no parent would believe their child's autism diagnosis reflected a fad or fashion in the changing "gestalt."

Having read through centuries of research, studies, and case histories, we believe we're seeing "a real change," as Frances puts it for us—the evidence for which is both autism's absence before 1930 and its massive increase beginning in the 1990s. If Frances, an intelligent professional who has had the independence to question much of psychiatric orthodoxy, took another look, he might realize that.

◆ ◆ ◆

We've heard from CDC officials that they first began to suspect an epidemic when they heard reports of increases in the mid-1990s.[176] This would make sense. The inflection point began in 1988–89. Average age of diagnosis was around four years of age, so the first signs would have emerged in the mid-90s.

But the report that first put the epidemic on the map came from the study we've already mentioned from California, the largest state and one that has been in the vanguard of many trends that spread across the nation. In 1999, the California Department of Developmental Services released a startling report.[177] Tracking the number of autism cases from 1987 to 1998 and using the narrow definition of autism, PDD/ autistic disorder, the report found a rapid rise in autism in the 1990s.

(Significantly, the criteria excluded both PDD/NOS and Asperger's, meaning the latter's inclusion in the 1994 DSM-IV did not impact the numbers. Nor did the alleged "fateful typo" George Washington University anthropologist Roy Richard Grinker and Silberman use to discount everything that came after, which we'll discuss shortly.)

The California increase took the DDS caseload of PDD/autistic disorder in raw numbers from 2,778 to 10,360, more than tripling in a decade. Breaking out the data by birth year showed a rise in the late 1980s but then a jump in the latter part of the period, 1989–91(the same timing the EPA later reported was underway worldwide).

And "autism" was not simply substituting for other diagnoses. As a percent of total DDS clients, autism rose from 4.9 to 9.4 percent. And critically, there was no similar increase in comparable categories: cerebral palsy, epilepsy, or mental retardation.

Here was strong evidence of a real increase in the most severe form of autism. It was swelling the department's caseload while other disorders were remaining static as a percentage of the total, suggesting this was not just a population increase or a relabeling of one of the other disorders as autism.

And it began well before the DSM-IV, whose inclusion of Asperger's was irrelevant to these California numbers anyway. The study was just the first snapshot, not a conclusive portrait, and it had its weaknesses. It didn't report prevalence or incidence rates, just numbers of cases being served by DDS. It included all ages, which meant a great deal of variation in the rate per age—three-year-olds would naturally be less fully diagnosed than eight year olds. And the increases, though large for the time, were modest relative to later reports.

Nonetheless, a credible report from a large state that found the rate of severe autism almost quadrupling in a decade with no obvious explanation made a big splash. That was in part because it confirmed what many were feeling—that there were simply a lot more cases of autism.

This was a direct challenge to autism orthodoxy—that autism was a genetic disorder that was not susceptible to the kind of sudden increase the California numbers showed. Not surprisingly, an orthodox response to this challenge popped up quickly.

In 2002, a team of researchers from Kaiser Permanente published a study[178] in the *Journal of Autism and Developmental Disorder (JADD)*, in which "the role of diagnostic substitution, trends in prevalence of mental retardation without autism were also investigated." The study compared rates of autism (full syndrome) and mental retardation in three- to ten-year-olds in California. The focus on rates was an improvement over the DDS report. And this time, the analysis found there *was* diagnostic substitution in California. If true, it was a blockbuster finding.

This took things back to the steady-state autism theory—an epidemic, if anything, of reclassification, not real cases. Eric Fombonne, a Canadian researcher who had done multiple studies that found little support for an increase in autism rates, praised the authors, crediting them for "carefully analyzing the California dataset."[179] Perhaps the "epidemic scare" would be over before it began.

Not so fast. One of us saw the study and realized the claim of diagnostic substitution underlying the increase in the initial study was wrong. The crucial realization was that, unlike the original DDS study that found the threefold increase, the reanalysis was comparing apples and oranges. Measuring trends in autism rates by comparing the number of three-year-olds who had entered the California system to the number of ten-year-olds made little sense when the average age at the time of diagnosis was between four and five: the trend would be driven by the most recent kids, the three-year-olds, for whom the rates would be far too low. Mark, a business analyst with a strong background in statistics but no previous publications on autism, shared his observations with a prominent epidemiologist and a neuroscientist. Both concurred, so the three of us wrote a commentary supporting the original finding of a real increase and challenging the new paper. We argued that mental retardation rates didn't go down (similar to the DDS finding) and autism rates should actually have risen faster than the Kaiser team reported. We submitted our paper to *JADD* within weeks of the original analysis.[180]

Soon, dramatic support for our position emerged. The MIND Institute at the University of California at Davis issued its own report.[181] First, it concluded the autism rate increases couldn't be explained by loosening of criteria. Second, there was no shifting of cases from mental retardation to autism—no diagnostic substitution—which was becoming the keystone arch keeping Epidemic Denial from collapsing in the face of the new California numbers.

We waited with eagerness to see if our rebuttal would have an impact. It took a few months for any response to come back from *JADD*, but in March of 2003, the authors of the first analysis claiming there was no real increase in autism published a stunning finding alongside the publication of our critique in *JADD*.[182] They admitted they were wrong. They calculated rates keeping age of ascertainment constant, and with that "apples to apples" approach, they found there was no diagnostic substitution in California. MR rates were, as we had argued, flat over the period. And after keeping age at assessment constant, there was a large and even steeper rise in the rate of autism cases.

Later that year, in what felt like definitive corroboration of an epidemic, the California Department of Developmental Services published an updated and improved version of their report.[183] This time, they reported prevalence rates and not just their caseload. These were now as high as thirty per ten thousand for kids born in the 1990s. (Remember Torrey's prospective study finding an analogous 4.7 per ten thousand rate in children born in the 1960s.) The study showed once again that age at diagnosis mattered, since rates by birth year increased when kids were young. And the study showed again there was no drop in MR; in fact, the caseload *increased,* slightly more than cerebral palsy and epilepsy.

Here is where Epidemic Denial goes to die. Diagnostic substitution, the last refuge of Gulliver in the modern age, doesn't provide a haven, either. We know from Torrey we weren't overlooking autism cases; we know from all kinds of corroborating studies that no one else was either, going way back in history; and we know from a careful examination of the timing and changes of the DSM-IV that it wasn't expanding criteria into a false sense of an epidemic, either.

This finding has proven durable. Although some studies have continued to claim US diagnostic substitution, even the most aggressive of these have never found it in California, the nation's largest state, with the most stringent apples-to-apples criteria and most road-tested methodology.

As the 2003 California reports emerged, another report from Minnesota confirmed the findings of no diagnostic substitution. A group from the University of Minnesota came out with an analysis of autism trends.[184] This study, by contrast to the narrow California criteria for autism, used the full autism spectrum as defined in DSM-IV, comparing ASD rates for a specific set of birth years (1989, 1991, and 1993). Crucially, they kept age constant for these calculations.

In the only published study reporting on ASD rates at the 1989–90 inflection point, the numbers rose sharply. For eight-year-olds (the standard age at assessment that was later adopted by the CDC), rates went from twenty per ten thousand in the 1989 birth year to thirty-five per ten thousand in 1991 and sixty-six per ten thousand in 1993. A tripling in just four years.

Like the California DDS studies, the Minnesota study also looked at the corresponding trend in MR diagnoses, which remained flat, as did rates for most other disabilities. Here it was again—another state level analysis with no evidence for diagnostic substitution between autism and MR.

Two states, same finding. But what about the nation as a whole? Shortly thereafter, the first national study came out.[185] The methodology was complicated but like the California and Minnesota studies, the authors again found no diagnostic substitution between autism and MR: "Because there was no indication of decreases in [the mental retardation and speech/language categories] concomitant with, and of similar magnitude to, increases in autism classification prevalence, these data do not support the hypothesis of diagnostic shifting."

In the meantime, a far broader project in autism surveillance, the CDC's ADDM—the Autism and Developmental Disabilities Monitoring network—was in the process of launching. The ADDM network first published autism rates in 2007 for children born in 1992.[186] But early outputs of the CDC's work were published before that, starting in Atlanta, the CDC's own backyard. In the early 1990s, the CDC began its work on MADDSP—Metropolitan Atlanta Developmental Disabilities Surveillance Program—first with cerebral palsy, mental retardation, and hearing and vision loss with data going back to the 1982 birth years and then with autism, which was tracked as far as 1986 birth years. The CDC's initial autism study was published in 2003—although with the same error as the Kaiser Permanente study, treating autism rates measured in three- and ten-year-year-olds as the same—reporting data from the 1986 to 1993 birth years. Like the California study that used a snapshot of three- to ten-year-olds, the first MADDSP[187] distorted the autism rates, making it look like autism rates went up and then down, when in fact metropolitan Atlanta was seeing the same autism increases California was. With respect to diagnostic substitution, this report added little and said nothing about any trend in the rates of mental retardation.

For over a decade, MADDSP was silent on diagnostic substitution. Then, to our surprise, the CDC quietly published a comparative report[188] with data on both MR and autism in 2015. It contained twenty years of MR data—tracing rates for two decades, from the 1982 to 2002 birth years, while also including autism data starting with the 1988 birth year. As with California and Minnesota, there was no evidence in the metropolitan Atlanta counties covered by MADDSP for diagnostic substitution. Autism rates rose from forty-two to one hundred fifty-five per ten thousand, almost quadrupling, while MR rates remained unchanged for the full two decades.

This study suppressed data that would have made the point even more emphatically, because the CDC had data on autism going back even further than 1988. If we add this data to the 2015 report (the 1986 and 1987 data on nine- and ten-year-olds, which was published in the 2003 MADDSP report on autism), then the rate in Atlanta started even

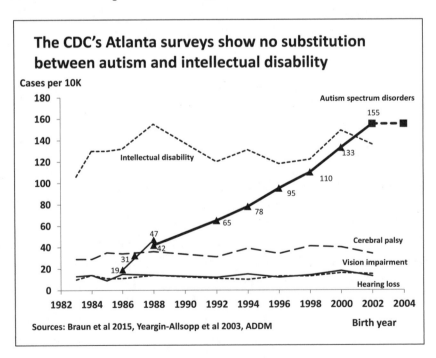

The CDC's Atlanta surveys show no substitution between autism and intellectual disability

Cases per 10K

Autism spectrum disorders

Intellectual disability

Cerebral palsy

Vision impairment

Hearing loss

155

133

110

95

78

65

47

42

31

19

Sources: Braun et al 2015, Yeargin-Allsopp et al 2003, ADDM

Birth year

lower than forty-two per ten thousand—at nineteen per ten thousand in 1986—giving an eightfold increase in autism in sixteen years. The full picture, combining the 2003 and 2015 studies, is shown on previous page.

So three states—California, Minnesota, and Georgia—and one national study reported no diagnostic substitution, confirming in multiple locations and in multiple studies that there was no reason to doubt the reality of the autism epidemic. But diagnostic substitution as a theory seems catlike in its ability to bounce back from the dead. A new author, Paul Shattuck, took another crack at the argument, alleging in a 2006 study[189] that diagnostic substitution still worked in the United States as a whole to explain the autism explosion, even if it didn't add up in the widely discussed and carefully calibrated California numbers. More recently, another group of authors from Penn State made a similar argument using the same database as Shattuck.

As we finalized this manuscript, one of us has submitted a detailed analysis for publication with University of Colorado scientist Cindy Nevison. This analysis uses the same data that Shattuck and the Penn State authors deploy. In contrast to their findings, this new analysis shows conclusive evidence that in a majority of states, the diagnostic substitution argument fails as badly as it did in California: in those states, the MR rate is flat or increasing, while the autism rate rises. In a small group of states, while it may be the case that the MR falls while the autism rates rise, there is little support for the idea that one is substituting for the other. (These states are mostly southern, represent only 15 percent of the population, and show odd and irregular trends in MR rates, but in an asymmetrical way and not in a way that appears to have anything to do with the rise of autism. Autism rates in these states actually rose more slowly than average!) Clearly, something else happened to MR rates in these states, not diagnostic substitution with autism. We hope that this analysis will put an end to the last leg of the stool of the Epidemic Deniers.

Our Bristling Contempt

In the almost three decades since autism cases began to spike, and the seventeen years since the first California numbers put statistical parameters around the increase, the efforts to explain it settled into two camps. Camp 1—ours—says the rise in rates is real. This book is an elaboration on that single idea. The rate was essentially zero until 1930; then something new happened to cause the first cases; then something more happened to cause the epidemic. We have tried to look for plausible hiding places for autism (Gulliver) before 1930 and listened to the best arguments against an increase since the 1990s: this chapter's discussion with Allen Frances and our analysis of Torrey, the best study ever done of autism rates between the discovery of autism and its explosion.

So while there is detail required in making our case—what was the rate of Heller's disease in 1930? How did the CDC count autism cases beginning in 1994?—our argument is simplicity itself, and we're happy to have it stand or fall based on readers' sense of how strongly we make the case. Essentially, we're applying Occam's Razor, the dictum named after the medieval theologian who said that the simplest explanation is usually correct. Of course, he didn't talk like that; what he actually said was that "entities must not be proliferated unnecessarily." And in fact he put it in Latin, so our maxim really reads this way: *entia non sunt multiplicanda praeter necessitate.*

One might say the theory with the least assumptions wins—at least it wins the first round. So if you have no autism, followed by a lot of autism, the assumption to look at (or rule out) first is that autism cases actually *did* begin at a given point, and *did* increase dramatically.

To argue otherwise requires more assumptions, as we've seen. Now, more assumptions don't necessarily mean this "no epidemic" theory is wrong—it could be true that autism cases were overlooked, then recognized, then wildly overdiagnosed. And as Einstein said, "Everything should be made as simple as possible, but not simpler."

We hope you agree with our method, our evidence, and our argument, but we still feel an obligation to lay out an array of counter-explanations that Deniers have deployed from time to time. Some of them are well-meaning speculation while some look like the worst kind of self-protective nonsense; in sum, they are the kind of "entities"—ideas, grand theories, claims with no evidence—that proliferate when the simplest explanation is set aside too quickly (and happens to be correct).

Let's group these lame excuses in a way that makes their common themes apparent. The first excuse is that you, dear reader, are in over your head when you try to put your own common sense against the "experts." We have a thing against that latter word and employ scare quotes liberally when we use it. "Experts" have blamed parents for causing autism; "experts" have blamed genes for causing autism; "experts" have blamed parents who witnessed vaccine reactions as being anti-vaccine (ignoring the fact they had fully vaccinated their child right on schedule); and "experts" have blamed people like us for wrapping all that in a ball of Silly Putty and stretching it into a ridiculous theory that there really is an autism epidemic.

You see, it's all very complex and methodological and you should leave the heavy statistical lifting to the social scientists. For instance, you say the rise in autism cases in California is significant? Well, Donvan and Zucker have some news for you: when there are more people, they demand more services.

"For example, demand for anything—from drivers' licenses to public playgrounds—could be expected to go up when a population increase is under way," they write in *A Different Key.*[190] Then, as they often do, they stomp all over their point. "Indeed, during the years covered by California's autism report, the population did get significantly bigger, by roughly 16 percent. That was a factor that an epidemiologist would need to take into account and possibly subtract from any overall trend in whatever he was measuring. It is not a complicated adjustment to make, and indeed, the team that produced the California numbers purposefully did not count children who had moved into the state during the years they were examining."

So first of all, California's counters *omitted* those who moved into the state—perhaps they were seeking better autism services or for some other unfathomable reason were skewing the numbers. And furthermore, while the population increased by 16 percent, including the out-of-state arrivals, the autism rate *tripled* during this period. Making this kind of argument shows that Donvan and Zucker, are, at heart, Deniers.

Moving right along, as they are so often keen to do, the authors noted "there were many other confounding factors that were not so easily corrected for, and none was more nettlesome than the lack of clarity about who should be counted in the first place." Oh, please. What lack of clarity? They counted the full-syndrome, autistic disorder kids. Stop with the "lack of clarity" argument already.

But maybe the whole thing is really just "diagnosis shopping," or parents pushing for an autism diagnosis because supposedly they'd get better school services, Donvan and Zucker suggest. Well, first of all, if there is nothing wrong with your child, why shop for any diagnosis—any label signifying disability at all? Ah, but "It was known anecdotally that pediatricians and other professionals who held the power to label occasionally tilted the scale in the evaluations to ensure a child's access to better programs and state services."[191] Once again, if true, "occasionally" tilting the scale toward an ASD diagnosis has nothing to do with the twentyfold increase we can see from the 1960s (Torrey) to today (the CDC and just about everyone else).

Frances also brought up diagnosis shopping in our back-and-forth in Orlando in September. Mark countered: "This is not something parents make up. When my daughter was diagnosed at two and a half years old, we were heartbroken. The notion that we were trying right off the bat to seek unneeded educational services, that's just nuts. That's just the time when autism is diagnosed. At three years old, parents are thinking about their kids going into pre-school. They're not trying to bilk the system for more services. That's an insult to say that when we receive a diagnosis on a manifestly disabled child who can't speak, is spinning in circles, and there are thousands and thousands, the notion that that's just health-care seeking behavior, that's an insult to the families."

But maybe the cases just piled up for many years before they were counted (diagnostic accretion). Or the DSM kept moving the goal-posts. Or maybe different ways of counting—by states or via school special service data. . . .

◆ ◆ ◆

Those claims at least have the virtue of being grounded in arguments that *might* be true. The second category is stuff that boggles the mind but gets trotted out by imposing-looking people. One is the "geek effect" that Silberman popularized with his 2001 *Wired* magazine piece, arguing that a supposed high rate of Asperger's in Silicon Valley came because previously unmarriageable—heck, undatable—males hooked on computer code and gaming suddenly had good incomes and nice cars and could attract babes—some of them similarly tilting toward the spectrum—and make babies. Simon Baron Cohen of Cambridge University, one of those imposing people we cited earlier, called this "assortative mating," a new pecking order in which the Sheldon Coopers of the world (he and his pals work at CalTech on *The Big Bang Theory)* are thrown together with the geeky Amy Farrah Fowlers. This would lead to geekiness squared, or at least doubled, in their offspring, which as we all know means autism on prime-time TV. (Can you feel our bristling contempt here?) This is essentially a "genetic epidemic" argument—a huge increase in one generation due to genes, not toxins—and fails the laugh test. One of us has called this contemptible idea "Geeks Get Lucky" and notes an equally ridiculous variant, "Geeks on the Go," where immigrant men find spouses who attribute their strangeness to cultural differences.

Joined at the hip with that folly is the one that suggests if you create an autism services industry you will create a lot of autism—the "build it and they will come" model transferred from *Field of Dreams* which, let's remember, was a fantasy wrapped inside a movie. If you build it they will come—*if* they have autism. We've noted before that early autism prevalence surveys occurred in states (like Wisconsin) and countries (like Japan) that were early leaders in autism prevalence. The higher numbers didn't occur because someone did a study; someone did a study because they sensed there were cases to be found.

Close behind is the Rain Man canard, in which the 1988 movie that brought attention to autism somehow made caregivers realize for the first time that they had a full-syndrome, completely disabled, "markedly and uniquely different child" on their hands. Here we are going to tell you a story that superficially seems to argue for the Rain Man effect. When one of us joined Bernard Rimland on a panel several years back at the Washington State Autism Society conference, Rimland introduced an autistic savant and put him through some amazing feats of calculation and memory. This man said he went to see *Rain Man* and, during a scene where Dustin Hoffman was asked to do a complex calculation, he shouted out the answer to the stunned theatergoers before

Hoffman himself did. On the way out, he touched the life-size poster of Hoffman and realized for the first time that he had the same disorder.

We don't doubt or wish to diminish the poignancy of that story. Of course it can happen that new attention to any phenomenon can make people aware of their own connection to it. That's one person, and good for him. One in a million.

Far more often, folks with zero claim to autism have decided it's fun or fitting to claim membership in the tribe. Jerry Seinfeld told the world in 2014 that he believes he falls on the autism spectrum "on a very drawn-out scale." He told Brian Williams: "You're never paying attention to the right things. Basic social engagement is really a struggle. I'm very literal. When people talk to me and they use expressions, I don't know what they're saying, but I don't think of it as dysfunctional. I just think of it as an alternate mindset."[192]

Within a couple of weeks, he took it back. "I don't have autism. I'm not on the spectrum," he told Billy Bush on *Access Hollywood*. "I just was watching this play about it and thought, 'Why am I relating to it?' I related to it on some level. That's all I was saying."[193]

Self-diagnosis may be the most vexing phenomenon contributing to Epidemic Denial. Advocates like James Carley, who we described in the introduction, give one the sense that the disorder is simply part of the diversity rainbow. Many argue against being considered disabled and bristle at words such as "recovery," "cure," or even "treatment," which might help ameliorate the more confining aspects of their condition. "Nothing about us without us," they say, an exemplary motto for inclusion—of themselves. They seem remarkably less interested in the severe cases who, by definition, are "without" the ability to participate in advocacy discussion, and for whom parents, and ultimately siblings and other committed lifetime caregivers, are the appropriate people to speak for the vast majority of people with autism who are vastly more disabled.

◆ ◆ ◆

And now, the "fateful typo." In 2007, Roy Richard Grinker, an anthropologist at George Washington University, wrote *Unstrange Minds*,[194] perhaps the first of the modern wave of Denier tracts for mainstream audiences. Grinker, an autism parent and fine writer, bore down on the epidemic claims by dissecting the series of DSMs over the years as if they were serial-murder victims, shot full of confusing language and shifting criteria by a perp with the seeming desire to create a false impression of more, and more, and more cases with each iteration.

As with Donvan and Zucker and Silberman and Offit, Grinker caught the attention of mainstream media, eager to debunk the epidemic argument with peculiar zeal (more on that in the next chapter). In an article in January 2007 with the unironic title "Is the Autism Epidemic a Myth?"[195] *Time* magazine's Claudia Wallis wrote:

"Epidemic is a powerful word. It generates bold headlines, congressional hearings, research dollars and dramatic, high-stakes hunts for culprits. It's a word that has lately been attached to autism. How else to account for the fact that a disorder that before 1990 was reported to affect just 4.7 out of every 10,000 American children now strikes 60 per 10,000, according to many estimates—the equivalent of 1 in 166 kids? [Now, a decade later, 1 in 68, or more than twice as many.]

"But what if there is no epidemic? What if the apparent explosion in autism numbers is simply the unforeseen result of shifting definitions, policy changes and increased awareness among parents, educators and doctors? That's what George Washington University anthropologist Roy Richard Grinker persuasively argues in a new book sure to generate controversy."

Grinker, Wallace wrote, attributed the "epidemic" to rising awareness, broader definitions in every DSM update, changes in school record keeping, more help and less stigma for those getting an autism diagnosis, and relabeling—what we've called diagnostic substitution.

We've taken our shot at all these, but Grinker's "typo" argument is worth spelling out as it shows the kind of pinhead dancing that results in "no epidemic" assertions the media adopts uncritically.

According to Grinker's description of the DSM-IV, "there was an error in the final manuscript. It is not well-known, even among experts, but in 1993, when the authors of the child psychiatry section of the DSM were editing the proofs of the new DSM-IV, which would be published in 1994, they missed a critical mistake. For PDD-NOS, the largest group of autism spectrum disorders, the authors had intended to write as the criteria, 'impairment in reciprocal social interaction and in verbal or nonverbal communication skills.' A different text was accidentally published. It said, 'impairment of reciprocal social interaction or verbal and nonverbal communication skills, or when stereotyped behavior, interests, and activities are present.' The authors had wanted someone to qualify as autistic only if they had impairment in more than one area, but the criteria, as published, required impairment."

They wrote "or" when they meant "and." Aha! In *NeuroTribes,* Silberman leapt on this supposedly major lapse: "This fateful typo went uncorrected for six years and was unacknowledged in the literature until the editor of the DSM-IV Text Revision, Michael First, finally copped to it in a notably understated article in an obscure journal in 2002. This certainly didn't mean that every child diagnosed with PDD-NOS in the years between 1994 and 2000 was misdiagnosed, but the impact of the botched language was potentially significant."[196]

There he goes again—insinuating First did his best to bury the mistake but also copping to the fact that it might not be a big deal at all. It was just *potentially* significant. Silberman and Grinker are gleeful that a reanalysis of some field tests with the typo corrected yielded fewer PDD/NOS cases, but as this wrinkle was smoothed out in the subsequent update, the epidemic was roaring along at full speed, smashing through anything that could be cooked up to explain it, from the addition of Asperger's to a tempest in a typo.

As Mark told Allen Frances in Orlando, this obsession with diagnostic criteria causing an epidemic is inside-baseball stuff that overlooks the reality of the epidemic and instead finds ever-proliferating ways to deny it: "The DSM-IV diagnostic criteria for autism were an improvement over the previous ones, and they were all consistent with each other, so it was actually representing what was going on in the world.

"The thing that happened was DSM-IV was implemented just in time to be blamed for a real increase in the condition that was valid and perceived everywhere including by the CDC. That's what they'll tell you—in the mid '90s we started to hear stories of increasing autism. It wasn't 'DSM-IV' autism, it was just more autism. And so the problem is that a real increase in autism is being excused by the DSM-IV. Which was a responsible project that you managed, and managed well."

◆ ◆ ◆

As we've made our way through the thicket of autism denial, we keep returning to first principles and simplest explanations, to Occam as opposed to Offit, to case studies and qualified observers as opposed to vague "anecdotes" that Donvan and Zucker and Silberman toss around like confetti at an autism benefit.

After the public session with Frances, Dan put to him the question with which we began the book—how his profession could have missed Goliath (autism) all this time and now believe he was always there. Dan tried the Heller-Weygandt test that makes Epidemic Denial not just implausible but, in our view, impossible.

Dan: "I'm interested that Heller-Weygandt disorder could have been precisely diagnosed even though it was so rare in the early 1900s, and yet no one talked about autism, which is similar and would have been occurring in just a slightly younger cohort. Do you think that's kind of odd?"

Frances: "One of the things is the history of psychiatry has been the history of different tides or fads. Different fads of looking at human distress. Human distress has always been there. The symptoms can be very similar over time but the descriptions of them and the way you categorize them can change dramatically. Suddenly . . . when there's a sudden increase in a diagnosis, to me that's a change in the way we see it and label rather than a change. You guys have exactly the opposite idea."

Dan: "We do. I think this may be an exception."

Frances: "That may be where we disagree; whether this is more appropriately determined at the moment we're seeing things this way—thirty years ago we were seeing them this way—and the change, the shift in gestalt can be explained by a shift in gestalt or a real change.

"I'm seeing the shift in gestalt and you guys are seeing the change."

◆ ◆ ◆

Well said. We *are* seeing the change. Heller-Weygandt is not a fad or a shift in gestalt, and neither is the Gulliver of this generation of childhood disability: autism.

Who benefits from this absurd idea?

CHAPTER 7

The Dynamics of Denial

"It is very hard to learn from very big mistakes."
—Karl Popper, *"The Poverty of Historicism"*[197]

The only-too-real rise in autism carries with it the imperative for action. Yet denial stands directly in the way of all of our society's corrective mechanisms. Epidemic Denial and Epidemic Doubt, which are members of the same inertial species, hold back this moment of truth—indefinitely and irresponsibly.

Leading Epidemic Deniers such as Silberman, Donvan, and Zucker have created elaborate constructs that block these corrective actions. They distort some appealing notions: *awareness*—because we were supposedly so blind for so long; *acceptance*—because autism is an identity that has been mistreated for too long; and *inclusion*—because all of the rest of us must be instructed how to live up to our responsibilities to this identity group. They're wrong.

All of us can agree that accepting this new autistic population is critically important. But if we refuse the awareness that it is, in fact, a *new* population, our acceptance will be clumsy and ineffective. It's one thing to accept a population that has already been with us; it's quite another to accept a tsunami—a newly affected population numbering in the millions. The challenge of inclusion is deeply affected by the same contrast. Inclusion is simply an act of respect to a preexisting group; including a tsunami. While it is desirable, it is extraordinarily difficult, so, we shouldn't be naïve about the enormity of the task, especially in terms of the social costs involved.

The problems of these Deniers' constructs are moral as well as economic. They don't heal lifelong injury or ameliorate its devastating costs and consequences, and they don't keep even one child from subsequently being injured. The magnitude of the devastation is so grim that it triggers the natural impulse to look for the silver lining or the atypical success story. The damage involved in the epidemic doesn't lend itself to sappy evening news featurettes. It's so much more convenient to celebrate our inclusiveness once the damage is done. There is an entire industry of celebrities and nonprofits and feature writers and pharma-funded TV shows and "expert" doctors and scientists ready to empathize, exhort, and explain it all to us before moving on to the next colored-ribbon cause.

This gauzy feel-good gestalt is nowhere near good enough when a historic epidemic is unfolding day by day, child by child, here and now in the most advanced country on earth. As Jim Carrey put it with pithy brilliance on CNN's Larry King: "The *problem* is the problem."[198]

To understand how this problem—the unchecked epidemic, not the ancillary issues that come with it—continues, the first question we need to ask is the inevitable one of self-interest: *Cui bono?* Who benefits from this unconscionable failure to admit and address the simple truth? Given the magnitude of the autism problem, it's not surprising that powerful interests would look for ways to avoid being blamed for the problem, and even worse being held accountable in some fashion—financial or otherwise. As we wrote in the book's first sentence, trillions of dollars are at stake, including billions in profit, stock prices, bonuses, and liability. The dollar signs associated with the epidemic are so large that it's worth billions for the prime suspects to evade accountability.

So obviously, there are plenty of economic reasons to short-circuit the hunt for causation by pushing the false notion that there simply is no epidemic, nothing to see here. But there's an even deeper motivation for denial at work: The autism epidemic is so catastrophic—such a "big mistake," to use Popper's term—that both individually and collectively deeper interests are at stake. This man-made epidemic touches more than just money—it affects the view we have of ourselves as living in a good society, where good things happen to good people who play by the rules, where no one would possibly make as big a blunder as this and then try to make it go away, where no free press would allow the suppression of such an idea, and where good guys always win in the end. We like to think life is like a Hollywood movie. Some heroic figure or group will surely stand up and fight the good fight to its obligatory happy ending.

We are reminded of the W. H. Auden poem, *The Unknown Citizen*, written in 1939 and foreshadowing Orwell's famous *1984*. Auden writes from the perspective of the state apparatus charged with assessing the life of one of its citizens who recently died. This "unknown citizen" did everything right by the state's standards. He raised the right number of kids (five); he hated war but fought when called; he was hospitalized once but cured. Wrote Auden: "The Press are convinced that he bought a paper every day/And that his reaction to advertisements were normal in every way." The last couplet is the killer:

Was he free? Was he happy? The question is absurd/
Had anything been wrong, we should certainly have heard.[199]

If anything as grotesquely wrong as the disabling lifetime injury of roughly 2 percent of our children had been going on for a quarter century, we should certainly have heard. Some brave soul would have spoken up and have been followed by others. Instead, we hear nothing official except silence and denial, a broad institutional failure. This failure works in many ways. Most disturbing is the refusal to take the affected families seriously, especially the witnesses to injuries—mothers and fathers—in favor of offering sweet nothings about how love and a sense of community can make their lives better. The suppression of powerful concerns about the plausible environmental suspects—including vaccines and related toxins like pesticides—illustrates the distortions in the force field of scientific progress brought on by Epidemic Denial.

Who Benefits?

The people who benefit most from Autism Epidemic Denial are those who make the toxins and orchestrate the exposures that, however inadvertently, have caused the epidemic. They benefit, it should not be necessary to say, first by making money and then by avoiding culpability in the forms of legal, financial, and possibly even criminal liability. Putting out a product that causes widespread harm can kill corporations, who have no more wish to die or diminish than you and me—ask Johns Manville, which was a member of the Dow Jones Industrial Average of thirty stocks as late as 1982 but filed for bankruptcy under the deluge of lawsuits for cancer-causing asbestos. It now exists as the Manville Trust, whose sole purpose is to pay claims for maiming and killings its workers.[200] Major international corporations have rings of defenses and phalanxes of lobbyists and lawyers to anticipate and prevent every possible negative outcome. We do not. But to take the most prominent and controversial suspect, if vaccines proved to be a major driving cause of the autism epidemic, business and government entities would be existentially threatened and the media's credibility, already as low as 5 percent in a post-presidential election poll, would flirt with negative numbers.

So of course those who brought us the autism epidemic benefit the most by making sure everyone ignores the implications and by understating the real suffering of most people with autism and their families.

But what are those toxins and how are children exposed to them? This has become a question fraught with such anger and anguish that it may make sense to step back a bit and look at the current mainstream consensus—that autism is genetic, and hence not epidemic, though perhaps with vague environmental "triggers" in some cases—and then review the most plausible alternatives that do fit with the epidemic theory we embrace.

Epidemic Denial is, of course, the handmaiden of the genetic paradigm. Alas, the Deniers sigh, a certain percentage of the population will be born with certain genetic anomalies. Some are simple and easy to spot, both externally and in the body. Down syndrome comes to mind. Under the microscope, it's a simple but life-shaping chromosomal variation, a trisomy 21. Others take time to manifest, like Huntington's disease, which results in the death of brain cells but can take decades to kill the individual. Huntington's is often cited to argue that just because many cases of autism are now regressive—they follow a pattern of normal development in early infancy before manifesting by age three—that doesn't mean they aren't genetic. That would be more interesting if Huntington's suddenly affected one in sixty-eight Americans instead of five to seven in one hundred thousand, ten times less than Torrey and colleagues determined as the autism rate in the early 1960s.

Wikipedia, that collective font of wisdom that rules the web, has an entry for one of us that says, "scientific research suggests that autism is a primarily genetic disorder and that reported increases are mainly due to changes in diagnostic practices."[201]

Our schools and special-ed classes are not filled to the brim with changes in diagnostic practices; our state adult services budgets are not swelling to the breaking point because Asperger's was added to the DSM in 1994, and our own commonsense observation of more autism in our families, among our neighbors and friends, and in popular culture are not better oversight. They are evidence of more cases of *autism*. Many more.

And while the reason for that rise is not the focus of this book, we do feel an obligation to look at the lineup of possible suspects that are the likeliest triggers for an environmental disorder. If our autism epidemic claim is correct, *something* is causing it. Well, comes the response, even if *something is*, there are eighty thousand man-made compounds surrounding us in this post-industrial age, "and most haven't been adequately tested for their effects on human health," according to the Natural Resources Defense Council.[202] "These chemicals lurk in everyday items: furniture, cosmetics, household cleaners, toys, even food." You could add your own list—chemicals in flame-retardant pajamas, plastic in baby bottles, even the chemicals in the receipt you're handed when you pay your bill at a restaurant or big-box store.

Keeping this list so large makes it hard to even begin looking for the environmental cause or causes of autism, and that's just fine with folks who have a sneaking suspicion—in some cases, more likely guilty knowledge—that their particular toxic contribution is part of the autism problem. So we're going to adopt a method we've already used in this book—putting up some fence posts to corral them long enough to take a closer look at what they might have in common.

Common sense tells us that the likeliest chemical causes would be the most ubiquitous, since autism rates, while they vary by state, are higher everywhere. And you'd want to focus first on compounds that fit the growth curve of autism. For example, diet soda, whatever its manifold problems, can just about be ruled out. It's been around long before the autism epidemic, kids don't drink it, and while there are ongoing debates about its health effects, plus or minus, it really does not need to be anywhere near the top of our list.

But that's the kind of nonsense the people in charge of finding out will spout. In an article on the vaccine theory of autism that ran in *The New York Times* in 2005, National Institute of Mental Health Director Thomas Insel said, "Is it cellphones? Ultrasound? Diet sodas? Every parent has a theory. At this point, we just don't know."[203]

How condescending. Insel, whose special brand of psychobabble (he now works for Google) made it hard to know if he thought there was an epidemic at all (he did before he didn't, or so it seems), leaves out the one possibility that almost every parent has at least considered and many have accepted—that autism is vaccine injury. Approximately zero-point-none of the autism parents we have heard from in the last fifteen years believes diet sodas caused it.

So you would think that when serious scientists approach the issue, they would attempt to compare the rising curve of the autism rate— and especially the hockey-stick spike that even an agency of the US government says began worldwide in 1988—with the exposure levels of other toxic substances that might have followed a similar trajectory, including, but not limited to, vaccines and their components.

You would think. But we're dealing with denial here, and what's really toxic is the way data is spun and suppressed to both hide the epidemic—because there is then no corresponding fault line of commercial product to correlate with it—and promote the least plausible suspects—genes, rain, highway traffic, maternal age, paternal age, paternal but not maternal age, diet soda, and so on.

For example, in 2010, Philip J. Landrigan of Mount Sinai School of Medicine published a review in *Current Opinion in Pediatrics* titled "What Causes Autism? Exploring the Environmental Contribution."[204] Well, that's promising. To ask what causes autism suggests the reader might be rewarded with some kind of answer, especially on the environmental side of the equation.

Landrigan's review takes note of genes but moves quickly to the environment. "Genetic factors—mutations, deletions, and copy number variants—are clearly implicated in causation of autism. However, they account for only a small fraction of cases, and do not easily explain key clinical and epidemiological features. This suggests that early environmental exposures also contribute. This review explores this hypothesis."

Landrigan notes that we're now more aware of the effect of toxins such as lead, alcohol, and methyl mercury (more on the last in a moment) on developing brains, and therefore more open to the environment as a factor in early onset disorders. Even more significantly, he says, we know that toxic substances, including medicines, can and do induce autism when the exposure occurs in early pregnancy—"thalidomide, misoprostol, and valproic acid; maternal rubella infection; and the organophosphate insecticide, chlorpyrifos." He then goes on to completely rule out vaccines.

After all this buildup promising an answer to what environmental factors might cause autism, we get the pitch: "Expanded research is needed into environmental causation of autism. Children today are surrounded by thousands of synthetic chemicals. Two hundred of them are neurotoxic in adult humans, and 1,000 more in laboratory models. Yet fewer than 20% of high-volume chemicals have been tested for neurodevelopmental toxicity. I propose a targeted discovery strategy focused on suspect chemicals, which combines expanded toxicological screening, neurobiological research and prospective epidemiological studies."

Ah yes, more research. But once again, epidemic skepticism, if not denial, makes that research less likely to help by not correlating toxins with the course of the epidemic. Or, in Marty Feldman's words, *What hump?* Landrigan continues: "The reported increase in prevalence of autism has triggered vigorous debate as to whether the trend reflects a true increase in incidence, or is merely a consequence of expansion in the definition of ASD and greater awareness, improved diagnosis and better reporting. This highly controversial question is not yet settled. A recent critical analysis concludes that increases in recognition, changed diagnostic criteria, and changing public attitudes about autism have played a major role in catalyzing the upward trend in reported prevalence. This analysis observes, however, that the possibility of a true rise in incidence cannot be excluded."

This is the Donvan and Zucker gestalt—there might not *not* be an epidemic: there might really be one! That is hardly a game-changing observation. Landrigan, who heads the Children's Environmental Health Center at Mount Sinai, did offer ten chemicals he considers to be leading contenders for causing autism and other environmental disabilities:

1. Lead
2. Methylmercury
3. PCBs
4. Organophosphate pesticides
5. Organochlorine pesticides
6. Endocrine disruptors
7. Automotive exhaust
8. Polycyclic aromatic hydrocarbons
9. Brominated flame retardants
10. Perfluorinated compounds

But here's where garbage in—lack of clarity over the very real increase in autism—produces garbage out: listing substances whose exposure levels have actually been *decreasing* in many cases since the autism epidemic began. If lead were going to trigger an autism epidemic, that epidemic would have come and possibly gone—leaded gasoline was phased out of use in gasoline starting in 1973 and gone by the 1980s, years before autism rates began rising sharply. Number two on the list is methylmercury, to which exposure comes mostly from predatory fish such as swordfish and tuna that pregnant women increasingly avoid. And of course there's no mention of its close cousin, ethylmercury, the vaccine preservative that many parents blame for autism. While its overall use in the United States has also declined, the CDC recommends that all pregnant women and people older than six months get flu shots, many of which contain mercury. And the agency, shamefully, has refused to state a preference for the non-mercury version.

While at first glance promising, Landrigan's approach merely selects politically correct toxins for attention and leaves out the serious debates. A more thoroughgoing attempt to isolate environmental triggers would tackle the tough questions head on: it would compare the trend of plausible and increasing exposure levels to the trend in autism rates, treating the epidemic as the real phenomenon it is and looking for correlations that could explain its hockey-stick ascent.

Oh, wait, that serious analysis *has* been done. Cindy Nevison, an environmental scientist at the University of Colorado, produced a fascinating report in the journal *Environmental Health* in 2014, aptly titled "A Comparison of Temporal Trends in United States Autism Prevalence to Trends in Suspected Environmental Factors."[205]

Nevison, unlike the Deniers, accepts that the epidemic is real, and actively rules out toxins that make little sense if it is: "Around 75 to 80 percent of the tracked increase in autism since 1988 is due to an actual increase in the disorder rather than to changing diagnostic criteria. Most of the suspected environmental toxins examined have flat or decreasing temporal trends that correlate poorly to the rise in autism. Some, including lead, organochlorine pesticides and vehicular emissions, have strongly decreasing trends. Among the suspected toxins surveyed, polybrominated diphenyl ethers, aluminum adjuvants, and the herbicide glyphosate have increasing trends that correlate positively to the rise in autism."

Her conclusion: "Diagnosed autism prevalence has risen dramatically in the US over the last several decades and continued to trend upward as of birth year 2005. The increase is mainly real and has occurred mostly since the late 1980s. In contrast, children's exposure to most of the top ten toxic compounds [on Landrigan's list] has remained flat or decreased over this same time frame. Environmental factors with increasing temporal trends can help suggest hypotheses for drivers of autism that merit further investigation."

Nevison's data on exposure trends is even more interesting than the report's text conveys. In a supplemental information file that accompanies the main article, she provides a table with all the environmental factors considered, a table showing that the highest statistical connection between any individual substance and autism rates—its correlation coefficient—is with increasing doses of vaccination. Let's repeat that: The highest correlation between the rise in autism and any one environmental factor is the increasing number of doses of vaccines. Other highly correlated toxins include glyphosate—which appears to lag the epidemic sufficiently to rule it out as the primary factor though not necessarily as a later stage contributor—and PBDEs, a flame retardant used in children's pajamas.

So one of the very first hurdles we have to clear is to get past the continuing refusal to consider vaccines as a factor, despite the testimony of thousands of parents who say they witnessed immediate illness, regression, and subsequent autism diagnosis. This parental testimony is the heart of the vaccine argument. Accounts by thousands of our fellow citizens cannot be dismissed as confounding association with causation, looking for someone to blame or sue, or any other response but a serious and respectful effort to investigate such a significant number of near-identical observations. Someone who believes they saw their child develop autism as a result of following the vaccine schedule to the letter and tries to inform the medical profession, the media, and others is immediately branded an "activist," a "conspiracy theorist," or—as in Dan and Mark's case—members in good standing (nos. 29 and 306) of the Encyclopedia of American Loons, an online site devoted, ironically, to preserving solid science.[206]

The vaccine hurdle isn't the only one. The idea that *anything* manmade is a cause of autism is anathema to the previously mentioned phalanxes that guard the financial health of chemical companies, potentially to the disadvantage of our collective health. For example, take our old acquaintance Dr. Paul Offit, a vaccine developer with no standing in the autism world—he acknowledges never treating a single patient. Yet, as we've seen, he opines freely about the supposed absence of an autism epidemic, claiming that fifty years ago—the same era when van Krevelen was looking for a single case—there were really the same number of autistic children, just far fewer diagnoses.

Offit belongs to an odd outfit called the American Council on Science and Health (ACSH), where he and his colleagues swat away, like a noisome mosquito, any environmental evidence for autism causation. According to ACSH: "As science stood largely silent, Dr. Paul Offit—Chief of Infectious Diseases and the Director of the Vaccine Education Center at Children's Hospital of Philadelphia (CHOP) and long-time trustee and supporter of the American Council on Science and Health—took to the helm to fight the noble battle on behalf of children's health and safety."[207]

But it doesn't stop with vaccines. Any environmental link, especially one that involves exposure to neurotoxins, is nipped in the bud. In May 2016, following publication of a study suggesting a link with pesticides, it ran a blog post titled "3 Reasons Aerial Pesticides Are Not Causing Autism":[208] "There is no plausible biological mechanism for this correlation and none is proposed; it is simply two curves that happen to show an association, real or otherwise." Well, it's a free country, and if the ACSH wants to swat down pesticides—for which considerable evidence does exist of a biological mechanism and a role in neurological disorders including Parkinson's and autism—they are free to do so. It is worth pointing out that a *Mother Jones* investigation in 2013 reported that internal financial documents show that ACSH "depends heavily on funding from corporations that have a financial stake in the scientific debates it aims to shape."[209]

If denial is motivated largely by financial interests, though there may be multiple environmental suspects, the one at the top of the list for both controversy and correlation is vaccines. The question naturally arises: How much money is on the line in the development and distribution of vaccines, and how might that explain the motivations,

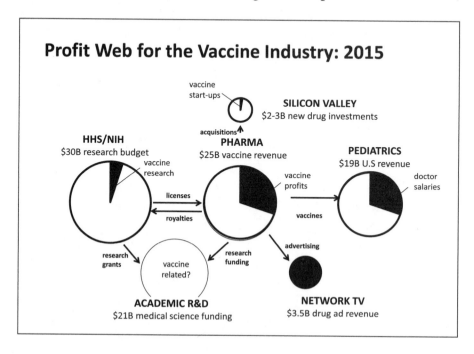

152

activities, and conduct of a wide variety of interested parties? The question *cui bono* in the vaccine business is a complex web of money, profits, grants, and quid pro quos. Describing the entire web that surrounds this "economy of influence" is too large a task for our purposes here, but a simpler treatment of the critical nodes in the profit web for vaccines is shown in the chart above.

As the saying goes, follow the money. Any search for the money trail in vaccines needs to start in one august and supposedly unimpeachable source of authority: The National Institutes of Health (NIH). In its own words—the largest funder of biomedical research in the world, the NIH controls more than money; it define the parameters of acceptable speech and investigation in the scientific community. No practicing scientist with career ambitions in mainstream science can afford to run afoul of its intellectual jurisdiction. NIH has both moral authority and market power—it is a monopsonistic buyer in the market for medical research. And while NIH may not have a profit interest (most of the time) in the outcomes of the scientific research, it has a clear institutional bias. An agency of the Department of Health and Human Services (HHS), NIH sits alongside its sister agencies, including the Food and Drug Administration (FDA), which licenses vaccines; the Centers for Disease Control and Prevention (CDC), which recommends and promotes them; and the Health Resources and Services Administration (HRSA), which negotiates compensation deals with the families of vaccine injury victims.

When science is proceeding in ways that have no bearing on its institutional partners, NIH can live up to its reputation as an arbiter of scientific quality and a force for progress. By contrast, when a scientific controversy such as autism and vaccines places an agency like the CDC squarely in the crosshairs of accountability, the NIH becomes an interested party. Expecting the NIH to act without prejudice in assessing the contribution of vaccines to the autism epidemic is like asking one presidential candidate whether the other is more qualified and expecting an objective answer.

NIH controls the purse strings for both autism and vaccine research. Autism received a paltry $200 million in 2015, a surprisingly small number in face of the largest epidemic of our time. Its spending on "vaccine-related research" dwarfed its autism investments at $1.6 billion.[210]

The NIH also has key links to other important players in the vaccine profit web. One little-known fact is that the NIH frequently files for patents on its vaccine-related research. When these patents protect research that yields successful commercial vaccines, NIH receives royalties from the pharmaceutical companies that bring these vaccines to market. One notable example: Merck's Gardasil vaccine sends millions of dollars in royalty payments to NIH every year.[211] Can NIH and HHS be expected to be objective about Gardasil's safety when they're a business partner with Merck? We think not.

NIH also provides an economic lifeline to America's leading research universities. Billions of dollars in taxpayer-funded research grants circulate throughout the academy every year. Despite the obligatory claims of academic freedom, most of these universities have become large-scale research businesses. Inside these hallowed halls, any dissident scientist with the temerity to challenge the government's position on a controversial question on the autism-vaccine question is putting his or her career at risk.

If the money trail starts with the NIH, the center of the vaccine-profit web is the vaccine manufacturers, major divisions within four of the world's leading pharmaceutical companies. Many years ago, the vaccine manufacturing industry was a very different animal. A highly fragmented industry largely populated by affiliates of local health departments and buoyed by only a handful of commercial products, the industry was a sleepy, low-growth, and low-profit business. Over the last several decades, that scenario has been transformed with the advent of the 1986 National Childhood Vaccine Injury Act. Vaccine makers now benefit from virtually complete liability protection against vaccine injuries, and since the late 1980s their revenues have exploded. By 2015, total industry revenue exceeded $25 billion, most of which flowed into the coffers of four global pharmaceutical giants—Merck, GlaxoSmithKline, Pfizer, and Sanofi-Aventis—all of them reporting vaccine sales of over $5 billion and profit margins, when disclosed, in the neighborhood of 30 percent.[212]

With pockets as deep as this, little exposure to product safety problems, and voracious ambition for growth, pharmaceutical money has pervasively lubricated the wheels of Denial. One example: Paul Offit, one of the more prominent autism Epidemic Deniers and defenders of the vaccine program, is a Merck-made millionaire.

Vaccine makers have customers, of course. In this case, the medical practices that purchase the bulk of the $25 billion vaccine revenues consist of the most sympathetic of all medical practitioners: the pediatrician. Everyone loves pediatricians. They take care of babies, don't they? Of course they do. But like every medical professional, pediatricians have a business to run, and the foundation of any modern pediatric practice is the most widely insured and acclaimed medical service there is: the well-baby visit.

New mothers, anxious to provide the best for their infant, are comforted by this ritual: the frequent presentation of their precious child to an expert who can reassure them that everything is fine and that their baby's development is on a healthy trajectory. Less well understood is that the well-baby visit has only one medical justification: the administration of vaccines.

As the vaccine schedule has exploded alongside the autism rate, so have the number of well-baby visits and the pediatric reimbursements that go along with them. It's not a stretch to say that the main *economic* function of a pediatrician is vaccine delivery.

The pediatric industry—the friendly face at the front line of the vaccine supply chain—is a $19 billion piece of the vaccine marketplace.[213] And America's pediatricians, all 28,660 of them, are a formidable corps of ambassadors. The largest single share of that $19 billion in revenue pays for pediatricians' salaries. To say that the livelihood of this doctor corps is dependent on the health and reputation of the vaccine business is no understatement.

◆ ◆ ◆

Other parts of the profit web are smaller than the main sequence of research, manufacturing, and delivery. But some of them are quite influential. The venture capital industry is one powerful community that has tied its wagon to the vaccine project. Venture capitalists invest in a wide range of start-up industries and in recent years venture capital has flowed heavily into the life sciences.

"Silicon Valley," common shorthand for the home of many prominent venture capitalists, has an economic interest in any breakthrough technology and has been eager to explore all kinds of new drugs and therapeutics, including vaccines. By one count, 271 vaccines are in the development pipeline.[214] Close to $3 billion per year in new venture capital has been flowing to the funding of novel drugs by venture-backed start-ups. Of this, vaccines make up only $60 million, but this clearly gives Silicon Valley skin in the game for the reputation and future growth of vaccines. Anything that puts obstacles in the way of new vaccine development inhibits their return on investment. Venture capitalists especially want to support the pharmaceutical companies' willingness to invest in vaccines, since offering their life sciences companies up for acquisition by a pharmaceutical company is a venture capitalist's primary exit strategy.

One of the earliest and most unusual participants in autism Epidemic Denial was *Wired* magazine, an odd nexus from which to enter into this debate. If one accepts that Silicon Valley is a player in the vaccine profit web, it's no surprise that a technology magazine like *Wired* would jump into the fray. Steve Silberman, late of *NeuroTribes*, is the *Wired* contributing editor who wrote the piece, "The Geek syndrome," in 2001.

Last but not least in the vaccine profit web is one of the major recipients of pharmaceutical advertising—television network news.

"After three months of viewing, I think I can say with confidence that the network evening newscasts are basically drug pushers for big pharma," Stephen King tweeted on November 9, 2015.[215] Horror writer King's comment may have been offhand, but much careful research has shown him to be dead-on. In 2005, *Columbia Journalism Review* tracked ABC, CBS, and NBC evening newscasts for a week in April; combining all three, sixteen ads for prescription drugs and eighteen over-the-counter drugs ran nightly, on average.

Early this year, we conducted our own survey along similar lines and found 44 percent of the ads on the evening network news are drug ads, with ABC leading the pack at 49 percent. It's likely that counted by minutes, the drug ads would stand out even more given that prescription drug ads need time for disclaimers.

Drug Ads on the Network Evening News	
	Total for the week of 1/9/17
NBC	
Total, excluding own show promotion	90
Prescription drugs	18
OTC	19
% drug ads	41.1%
ABC	
Total, excluding own show promotion	85
Prescription drugs	23
OTC	19
% drug ads	49.4%
CBS	
Total, excluding own show promotion	86
Prescription drugs	22
OTC	13
% drug ads	40.7%
All 3 networks	
Total, excluding own show promotion	*261*
Prescription drugs	*63*
OTC	*51*
% drug ads	*43.7%*

Of course, all this creates a massive conflict of interest—so large as to be invisible, like oxygen for humans and water for fish. White-coated solons like Paul Offit are greeted like Jonas Salk on the morning network shows. The fact that Offit has made millions from the vaccine program even while serving on the CDC's vaccine approval advisory board just doesn't seem to register.[216] Only the United States and New Zealand allow direct-to-consumer pharma ads, and even the American Medical Association has called for a halt;[217] it's really the media that craves the huge windfall. (When we raised the idea of ending pharma media advertising with a well-known former national news anchor, he replied: "What? Cut off the heroin?")

It's no wonder Big Media bows before Big Medicine. According to statnews.com, an online medical site, "Even as politicians and physicians press for strict limits on prescription drug ads, the pharmaceutical industry is pouring billions into new TV and print campaigns. Ad spending soared more than 60 percent in the last four years, hitting $5.2 billion last year. And there's no sign it's slowing. On the contrary: Nine prescription drugs are on pace to break $100 million worth of TV ad time this year.

We know from several sources that the pressure from pharma advertisers is relentless. Robert F. Kennedy Jr. said the following:

"I ate breakfast last week with the president of a network news division and he told me that during non-election years, 70% of the advertising revenues for his news division come from pharmaceutical ads. And if you go on TV any night and watch the network news, you'll see they become just a vehicle for selling pharmaceuticals. He also told me that he would fire a host who brought onto his station a guest who lost him a pharmaceutical account."[218]

Sharyl Attkisson, former CBC Washington investigative correspondent who now has her own independent program, knows that pressure firsthand. She described to us being called on the carpet after pharmaceutical sponsors complained about her reporting on the "discredited" vaccine theory of autism.[219]

The *Columbia Journalism Review* (*CJR*) took on the topic in 2005:[220] "There is a very real fear that taking the thimerosal theory seriously will prompt antivaccine blowback. Myron Levin, the *Los Angeles Times* reporter, said that some journalists have been cowed by the notion that 'by the mere act of covering this, they will instill panic in the vaccination-getting public, or feed mindless phobias that cause people to refuse to let their kids get shots.' That concern is reflected in the coverage and has implications for how deeply the story is reported. 'I think many news organizations have held back and given the story short shrift,' Levin said."

CJR itself was not immune from internal denunciation. As the efforts to turn Andrew Wakefield from an incompetent to an outright "fraud" (in the words of the *British Medical Journal*) proved successful, many media sources backpedaled furiously from even the appearance of impartial journalism. In 2013, the *CJR* published its first large article since the reasonably evenhanded 2005 piece on the vaccine controversy, this time titled "Sticking With the Truth—How 'Balanced Coverage' Helped Sustain the Bogus Claim that Childhood Vaccines

Can Cause Autism,"[221] and cited one of us at length as part of the bogusness. It went after its own report from 2007:

"*CJR*, too, played a role in sustaining the vaccine story. In a 2005 piece, Daniel Schulman, who's now an editor at *Mother Jones*, advised that it was 'too soon for the press to shut the door on the debate' about vaccines and thimerosal."

The use of the word "former" and "now with" pops up a lot in accounts of media coverage. One of us is a former wire service reporter who was let go the week after his first appearance on national TV about autism. In a C-SPAN interview about the vaccine controversy, Dan asked rhetorically: "Are all these parents who say their child had a vaccine reaction, got sick and immediately developed autism simply wrong? I don't think so."

"I don't think so" is not the way a zealot talks, it's the way a journalist familiar with a topic who has interviewed dozens of parents adds analysis to straight reporting. But it simply isn't tolerated today. At *The New York Times,* treating the idea that the mercury in vaccines causes autism seriously is expressly forbidden. "No false balance here," their ombudsman said in regard to complaints about suppressing that point of view.

◆ ◆ ◆

Cui bono? Most blatantly, those who benefit are those in medicine and the media with a symbiotic relationship built on deep, profound but often invisible conflicts of interest and heaps of cash. Their safest route is to be antagonistic or at least agnostic to the very idea of an epidemic increase. "What Epidemic?" as *Time* asked. "What hump?" asked Igor.

Who Believes?

It's not enough just to point to conflicts of interest that constrain the discussion of the autism epidemic and its concomitant environmental roots. More than simple conflicts and interests, issues of belief and ideology pervade the Epidemic Denier worldview. At its core may simply be a felt sensation that nothing this bad—the poisoning of a generation—or more—of children in an age of consumer safeguards, regulatory precautions, and a generally cleaner environment—could happen on our collective watch.

Karl Popper, the influential Viennese philosopher whose epigraph begins this chapter, speaks of the "poverty of historicism," in which Utopian thinking can lead to mistakes that are very hard to catch and correct before they wreak havoc (the bigger the mistake, the harder to catch).

"Every attempt at planning on a very large scale is an undertaking which must cause considerable inconvenience to many people, to put it mildly, and over a considerable span of time," Popper writes.

> Accordingly there will always be a tendency to oppose the plan, and to complain about it. To many of these complaints the Utopian engineer will have to turn a deaf ear if he wishes to get anywhere at all; in fact, it will be part of his business to suppress unreasonable objections.
>
> But with them he must invariably suppress reasonable criticism too. And the mere fact that expressions of dissatisfaction will have to be curbed reduces even the most enthusiastic expression of satisfaction to insignificance. Thus it will be difficult to ascertain the facts—i.e., the repercussions of the plan on the individual citizen; and without these facts scientific criticism is impossible.[222]

Utopian visions create far worse outcomes than those that emerge in the rough and tumble of an open society (the phrase for which Popper is justly famous), because it takes an authoritarian and utilitarian mind-set to create a "Utopia." "Making it difficult to ascertain the facts" and "suppressing reasonable arguments" could serve as the motto of Autism Epidemic Denial. We see two major Utopian threads of thought.

The first of these is the political idea often described as progressivism, which came out of the early twentieth-century reaction (led by Teddy Roosevelt) to the robber barons and asserted that government had a role in leveling the playing field by, for example, breaking up the trusts or establishing the national park system—that in some cases only big government could do big things. A generation later,

Social Security followed, and one generation after that, Medicare and Medicaid came along. Over time, as often happens with the pendulum swing of political ideas in America, progressivism reached an extreme that might be called the impulse of those in power to "fix" everything that could be fixed. Poverty could be fixed by public housing and welfare; health inequalities could be fixed by universal health care; and failure to reach every child with a good education could be fixed by kindergarten, then Head Start, then preschool, all of it funded or in other ways encouraged by government itself.

Thus, progressivism swung from the idea that some problems are so big that only government can fix them to the idea that big government can fix just about every problem and, in the most extreme instances, that resistance to the helpful hand of government is futile and might put you in harm's way.

Nowhere has this become more evident than in health care, and nowhere in health care more evident than the vaccination program, which began with attempts to wipe out a handful of deadly diseases that killed thousands of children every year (diphtheria, smallpox, eventually polio), an effort in which parents eagerly participated. Now that has morphed into a state-driven set of mandates that are becoming increasingly inflexible and invoke more and more draconian measures—no shots, no school; no flu shot, no job at the hospital; no personal or even religious exemptions; no consideration for whether a disease is deadly or even still in circulation; and no allowance for the rights of parents to decide these issues for themselves.

With the advent of liability protection for the drugmakers, the impulse to create more and more vaccines merged with the progressive impulse to impose the supposed benefits of modern health care on all. The free market, which America has relied on for years to sort out good products and ideas from bad, was essentially rendered inoperative in this most personal and invasive of marketplaces—the human body. This picture was mirrored in other aspects of society that caused the shock of the century in the political field, with Donald Trump elected president on a platform that might as well have been, "Tell the experts to go to hell."

Worldwide, Brexit sent the same message, and more shocks are probably coming. It is inevitable that this revolt will reverberate in the

161

autism world; indeed, even before Trump was elected, it already had. Trump asked Robert Kennedy Jr. to head a new commission to study vaccine safety. Though clarifications and uncertainties followed, it was clear that Trump—who has said too many vaccines too soon cause autism, a view we share—is intent on upending the top-down status quo when it comes to vaccination, just as he is with other topics.

The second of these Utopian threads is the faith in the technological progress that has driven much of our society, along with the confidence that the medical industry shares that momentum. From its perch in the high tower of expertise and assumed authority, the medical industry has long dominated the narrative about how medicine cures disease and eases human suffering. Recently, the public image of medicine has also become closely tied to technology. Channeling a broader belief in the march of technology, medicine has projected a sense of competence and confidence: that the inexorable march of human knowledge is saving lives and extending the human life span. As Moore's Law is at work driving exponential increases in computing power, so too goes modern medicine.

In reality, however, this "technological positivism"—the belief that human health will get better and better because machines will make it so—is a species of Utopian folly. The true nature of medical progress has followed a far less monotonic trajectory than transistor density on silicon. Medical technology is different from computing technology. Real breakthrough cures for major human diseases have come infrequently. The most important of these breakthroughs came long ago and in ways that belie the narrative of technological positivism. The invention of penicillin by Alexander Fleming in 1928 spawned the era of antibiotics, the single most important medical treatment breakthrough in human history. Within a few short years, the scourge of syphilis was erased; no other single therapeutic invention before or since has had so immediate and profound a benefit as this miracle cure. Far from a tale of linear innovation, perhaps the most interesting feature of the invention of penicillin was why it took so long to discover when the tool required for its discovery had been available for decades.

The evolution of an effective vaccine for preventing smallpox was another historic breakthrough. First promulgated by Edward Jenner, the vaccine that was based on the vaccinia virus eventually eliminated the threat of a disease that had killed and scarred millions and wiped the virus from the face of the earth. Unlike penicillin, the smallpox vaccine took centuries to attain its success, while the impurities in its preparation harmed and killed many. Although it was eventually successful, one of the most interesting features of the "smallpox vaccine" is the mystery of its true provenance: no one can pinpoint today where the active ingredient, the vaccinia virus, actually came from or how it was developed. Similarly, Ignatz Semmelweis's insight that protecting patients from germs in hospitals could be accomplished by the simple act of washing hands saved millions of lives, along with the associated philosophy of aseptic surgery ushered in the age of surgery (yet Semmelweis was ignored and ostracized for his discovery).

Technological positivism doesn't work well in explaining these most iconic medical breakthroughs. Unlike the physics of semiconductors and lasers, there are important limits to medical progress. There is No Moore (i.e., there are diminishing returns to medical interventions, not increasing returns, as with Moore's Law for information technology); and increasing dosage rarely increases effectiveness. Further, there are inevitably unintended consequences—for example, the rise in adult shingles incidence subsequent to increased varicella vaccination in childhood and the rising risk of mumps complications with vaccine failures. Most importantly, because we are dealing with biology and not physics, nature fights back when "cures" are overused: consider the rise in atypical pertussis infection, the spread of MRSA, and the difficulty in developing a durable vaccine against common influenza. Not surprisingly, unlike the dramatic successes of R&D investments in computing and telecommunications, there is a well-known pharma R&D crisis. Despite constant hype, medical technology has struggled to churn out new therapeutic inventions; as R&D spending has exploded, the rate of discovery has stagnated, with little hope for a revival.

Yet the power of the medical industry to indoctrinate its apprentices is powerfully evident in the durability of the myths every medical student is taught. Among these is the idea that "hospitals are safe places." Until the discovery of germ theory in the late nineteenth century, a hospital was generally a place where sick people went to die. Today, while the advances in surgery enabled by antibiotics and anesthetics can and do save lives, hospitals remain dangerous places. Hospital accidents, drug errors, and infections such as MRSA are among the highest causes of death. Another commonly held myth, "Germs are bad for us," has recently come in for a reckoning. While a handful of lethal microbes (e.g., smallpox, tetanus, Ebola) are always dangerous, we are learning that humans have evolved and thrived in symbiosis with germs. Our bodies teem with bacteria, and viruses are ever-present.

The dirty little secret of medical technology has been its focus on perverse and profitable blockbusters with little, if any, benefit in reducing disease and mortality. None of them qualify as cures and many of them are dangerous. Viagra is a recreational drug marketed as a treatment for a rare disease. Lipitor earns billions by providing marginal improvements to an indirect benefit (cholesterol reduction) that improves health outcomes (heart attacks) only modestly via a disputed mechanism (arterial plaque reduction). Lariam is drug designed as a preventive measure against malaria infection, but has a terrible safety profile. Gardasil, designed to prevent cervical cancers many years in the making, only protects against a handful of HPV strains, causes serious adverse events, including death, and provides no effective substitute for Pap smears.

This all may seem a little bit abstract, but Epidemic Deniers are motivated by more than just money. There is an implicit historicism—a belief that the future is always on a path to improvement—that underlies the resistance of so many to the idea that we have made so many children sick. Progressivism is founded on the idea of government intervention. The possibility that some of the most acclaimed government programs might have had unintended and catastrophic consequences is unthinkable.

Technology enthusiasts like to bundle medical technology with information technology under a shared rubric of technological positivism. But medical progress is dependent on the understanding of health and disease. When our understanding is poor, the technology will not work as intended. It will cause more disease and cost more money. With respect to medicine, adding more intervention is rarely the answer; understanding the nature of disease is the only way. With respect to government, adding more intervention can often bring poor performance, corruption, and even unchecked evil. One reason

Epidemic Denial is thriving is because true believers in these Utopian visions of progress cannot accept the reality of such a big mistake—the reality of autism.

Who Fights Back?

Against this tide, is there any effective strategy for facing reality and stopping the momentum for Denial? Paid trolls attack any online commentary raising questions about vaccines and autism. "Access journalism"—in which the all-important big interview or inside story depends on friendly relations with sources in key power centers—corrupts honest reporting. One example? In the egregious June 25, 2005, *New York Times* piece on "parents versus science" in the thimerosal controversy,[223] former CDC director Julie Gerberding has a single quote: "There's no conspiracy here." Most news outlets would (a) not be able to get an interview with Gerberding, and (b) if they did, would use far more than one quote, given the rarity of the encounter. To the *Times*, access is just business as usual. (As it turned out, there *is* an ongoing conspiracy at the CDC involving the suppression of higher autism rates in many children who received the MMR before age three.)[224]

So advocacy for an autism epidemic, with its environmental implications, is almost defined by a sense of frustration and rolling failure—both of us know the feeling, shall we say. But new energy has recently permeated the autism activist community. Two powerful movies helped the cause. First came *Trace Amounts,* by Eric Gladen, who was vaccine injured as an adult by a tetanus shot and was able to describe in vivid detail the consequences, which were mostly awful but also included an interesting side effect. Gladen, an engineer, was able to read and grasp blueprints and building plans in a flash, far more quickly and thoroughly than ever before. But he said the "gift," which faded as his overall health improved, was not worth the profound and even suicidal depression that accompanied it. His may be one of the better descriptions we'll ever get of an Asperger's-like mind-set. Other cases of injury leading to savant qualities—such as an average Joe who got mugged outside a pub and became a math whiz overnight—make clear that in many cases the "gift" of a highly specialized aptitude is itself a kind of injury to the brain's normal functioning—and slight compensation for the deficits that accompany it.

The second movie, *Vaxxed*, caused a revolution in the autism advocacy community. Made by Andrew Wakefield and professional TV producer Del Bigtree, it told the story of Dr. William Thompson, a CDC senior scientist who in a series of recorded phone conversations told scientist Brian Hooker that the CDC had fraudulently manipulated data on a key MMR vaccine safety study to hide a higher risk of autism for black boys who got the shot before three years of age—and for children in general who had no other serious conditions ("isolated" autism). Actor Robert DeNiro slated the film for the prestigious TriBeCa film festival, then withdrew it under pressure—grudgingly. But in the best of all possible outcomes for vaccine safety advocates, he went on the *Today* show and said everyone should view it, that his wife thinks their own autistic child was vaccine damaged by the MMR, and that "something's there" in the autism-vaccine connection.[225] The publicity sent the movie and its sponsors on a national bus tour that made masterful use of social media and may have created a tipping point in the outlook for the vaccine injury community.

Suppress the truth at your long-term peril.

◆ ◆ ◆

The election of Donald Trump as president creates an even larger opening for the acknowledgment of the epidemic—and its environmental roots. He has long tweeted—his preferred style of statecraft—that too many vaccines given too early and at the same time can cause autism. A critical side note on the 2016 presidential election: Regardless of one's political affiliation, if Hillary Clinton had won, the issue would have been dead for at least another four years. In a recent book—*A Brick Wall: How a Boy With No Words Spoke to the World*—on her autism experiences in Brick Township, New Jersey, autism parent Bobby Gallagher wrote that the publication of a study that found the world's highest rate of autism recorded up to that date was delayed because of Clinton. "Hillary [Clinton] is deciding on a run for Senate in New York, and you know how political these things can get," Gallagher says a CDC official told her. Apparently, the debate was over whether the word "high" to describe the rate was too incendiary for then-HHS Secretary Donna Shalala; when the report was finally published in 2001, the word was changed to "elevated," Gallagher said.[226]

Gallagher was baffled by the whole discussion, but the possible link between vaccines and the rising autism rate, which may have explained the rise in Brick Township, could have had implications for Clinton, who strongly backed vaccine development and expansion. Beyond the wording change, the data was presented in such a way as to obscure the increase. Gallagher says: "We would later discover that the numbers weren't changed, but they were certainly manipulated" to suppress the evidence of an increase.[227]

Autism advocates hope and expect that the environmental roots of autism, with a focus on vaccine injury, will be a priority for Trump and his administration. It is hard to overstate the fact that after years of begging and pleading for perfunctory meetings with lower-level staffers, with a brief duck-in by the Congressman or HHS or NIH factotum, who promises to have his staff follow up and disappears forever, the person in the Oval Office is now by all objective measures an ally, and one who is unlikely to renege (as George W. Bush did when he promised during the campaign to get rid of thimerosal).[228] Broadly stated, Trump has endorsed our view—more significantly, he has endorsed the view of Bernie Rimland when he called the Epidemic Deniers "Baghdad Bobs."

But perhaps as important as Trump himself is the era we appear to have entered that some have called "anti-globalist." People around the world are becoming sick of the "expert" gestalt, which creates a globally powerful, priestly class of unaccountable bureaucrats whose main role is to intermediate between The Truth and ordinary people, the latter group lacking in specialized knowledge but often possessed of infinitely greater Common Sense—including the sense to know they are getting a lousy deal, whether in terms of jobs or the autism that inexplicably disabled their child. A newspaper column cited "the tyrannical consensus of overpaid experts."

Brexit, the Trump victory, and other calls for greater local decision making—Frexit, Grexit, Calexit, et cetera—show the hold on power—which also means the hold on information, the hold on truth, the hold on the people's right to know and make the best-informed decision—may be slipping. With that trend could come a flood of information that totally transforms the autism world—confirming an epidemic, showing the role of toxins and perhaps vaccines in particular, and moving beyond the "expert" generation that perpetuated both the epidemic and its own priestly status in medicine, the media, and government.

Or not. We have learned to regard "breakthroughs" and "big moments" with skepticism. But the simple truth is that self-described conservatives, usually Republicans, with a focus on liberty, freedom, and localization of choice, have been far better allies than "progressive" Democrats over the past decade in particular. Some Democrats have been courageously outspoken—notably Robert F. Kennedy Jr., who ridicules the CDC as a "cesspool of corruption" and Paul Offit as a "biostitute, and San Antonio's State's attorney Nico LaHood, who joined a *Vaxxed* event to say he had seen his son descend into autism after a vaccination.[229] LaHood got the full "kook" treatment, as if what he was reporting from personal experience was somehow nothing but a political act or the benefit of received wisdom from anti-vaccine activists. LaHood and others contemplating public comment know by now that if Jesus Himself said vaccines cause autism, he would be relegated to his former status of itinerant carpenter who spent too much time in the desert.

These views are not meant to be partisan—Mark is a libertarian-leaning Republican, and Dan remains a classic liberal in the widest sense of the word. Both libertarian and liberal derive from *liberty*, which, in a word, shows us the way forward. A disorder first observed in a world of top-down "expert" hierarchy—that first blamed parents, then genes, both mistaken—is being confronted today with tools like the Internet that make suppression of the truth harder and harder—though not impossible, as continued attempts to cleanse Facebook, Google, and other modern outlets of vaccine "misinformation" continue. Increasingly, we've had to deal with the wholesale capitulation of the media, which now lumps concerns about vaccines and similar environmental issues with a whole class of "conspiracy theories" that don't pass the bar to deserve coverage.

◆ ◆ ◆

Political activism hasn't waited for a sympathetic president. It has instead been afoot for years, as it became clear that compelling new evidence could not compete in the skewed marketplace of ideas with denial, diversion, and just plain cover-up. Those who believed in vaccine injury felt like they were arguing their case to a medical version of the O.J. Simpson jury.

In response, a number of parents—including one of us—in 2010 created the Canary Party and in 2014 the advocacy group Health Choice, of which both of us are board members. A good deal of our thinking about the way forward is embodied in the guiding principles of the Canary Party, from which we quote here: [230]

> In 2010, a group of parents of children who were suffering from neurological and autoimmune disorders, and who had been active for years in their efforts to get mainstream medicine to address the causes of, and find treatments for, their children's poor health, faced the realization that while they had been earnest in their engagement of both the private medical industry and government public health officials, the medical establishment was not working in good faith with them. They decided that if anything was to be done about the epidemic levels of childhood chronic illness in the US, it would have to be a result of real political pressure to clean up the corruption in the medical establishment that was allowing bad pharmaceuticals, bad medical practices and bad public health policy to assault human health on such a wide scale.
>
> They began talking with those injured by medicine in other ways, those concerned with parental rights, with lack of choices in health care options, with environmental pollution, with nutrition, and with the encroachment of the medical industrial complex on the basic rights of the individual to practice informed consent in medical care.
>
> In the spring of 2011, it became clear that waiting to do something was no longer an option. It was time to launch The Canary Party, because the medical establishment is not paying attention to the sick canaries in our society that are telling us that there are serious problems that need to be addressed, and that if they are not, we must expect that society will begin to suffer greater and

greater collapse as more and more people succumb to the diseases and disorders rampant today . . . .

Our principles:

In recent human history, mankind has created and witnessed unprecedented changes in the balance between nature and technology. With the advent of the industrial revolution, technological progress has led to profound improvements in human health and quality of life. Important benefits such as improved sanitation and clean water have combined to reduce human mortality and extend the life span. As we recognize these benefits, we also know that technology works best when it serves human needs and worst when it imposes new risks on human development, creating a greater distance between nature and man. Paradoxically, as we become more reliant on technology, we risk losing sight of the proper balance between the benefits and risks of progress, especially in those technologies that intervene most directly in human health.

In order to restore that balance, we must pursue a future based on a more natural vision of human health, happiness and development, one that focuses on wellness rather than disease. The definition of wellness that guides the healing professions should not be the absence of symptoms in the presence of medical intervention, but rather the pursuit of health without the need for drugs. Realizing this future will require a more natural approach to wellness, especially early in life, but also throughout the life span. To restore the proper balance of nature and technology, The Canary Party seeks to restore balance to our civil society.

We hold these principles to be self-evident:

- That awareness of the new man-made epidemics is the first requirement for ending them;
- That when complexity clouds our understanding of health crises, our moral imperative is to first do no harm;
- That the best measure of a safe environment is the total health and happiness of an individual human being;

- That the individual's right to choose or refuse medical interventions affecting them or their children must be defended;
- That true empowerment requires that the individual is accorded and assumes responsibility for their own health, happiness, and nutrition;
- That full access to the healing professions and to truthful information is essential to liberty;
- That when injuries occur as a consequence of institutional failure, the victims deserve justice;
- That the cause of justice is best served when our governing institutions are free from commercial interests;
- That a compassionate society has a duty to provide injured and otherwise disabled citizens with an opportunity for happiness and to treat them with dignity.

◆ ◆ ◆

So the way forward might better be described as the *ways* forward, involving political action; engaged journalism in new forms and outlets; parents' relentless demands that their child's suffering be acknowledged and understood; siblings ascension to adulthood and with it the ability to share their experience and shape a better world; and perhaps direct action—loving but confrontational civil disobedience like that of the civil rights movement, for example—or a mass opt-out of some vaccinations that thwarts the public health agenda until that agenda includes recognition of the autism epidemic and an urgent search for its cause.

Epilogue: Normalizing Autism

A new era arrived on September 24, 2007, when *The Big Bang Theory* debuted on CBS. It is hugely popular in both first-run and syndication—where the money pours in like a flashing Vegas slot machine dumping a billion dollars in quarters—and if you want to ask *cui bono* from autism, *The Big Bang Theory* is, in its own way, a big winner. "The series about lovable, math-obsessed nerds is by far the biggest comedy on television, as it has been each of its past six seasons," the online site *The Wrap* reported last year.[231] "After 205 episodes, that is nothing short of astonishing." More than 20 million watch it every week.

The main lovable nerd, Sheldon Cooper, is autistic without anyone saying so, as if not mentioning the diagnosis makes it impossible to criticize the character portrayal. It does not. Literal minded in the way autistic people are, and displaying the iconic disturbance of affective contact that makes his relationship with Amy Farrah Fowler a mine-field of hi-*larious* sitcom mix-ups and hys-*terical* mishaps, the show's producers and fans can laugh all they want, but are completely disingenuous to deny his autistic features.

NJ.com reported in 2009[232] that *Big Bang* creator Bill Prady "has been asked about this a lot, and the short version is that, while Sheldon's personality—which was based on computer programmers Prady worked with years ago, well before Asperger's (a form of autism) was as common a diagnosis as it is today—certainly has traits in common with people with Asperger's, he would feel uncomfortable labeling Sheldon as such."

Traits in common with those with Asperger's are fine to lampoon, but it's not OK to say it's Asperger's? We've spent this book arguing that a few traits do not make for a diagnosis, but this is the reverse—a cynical exercise in playing a character with an identifiable disorder for laughs while acting shocked, shocked that anyone thinks it's autism.

"In the writers' minds, calling it Asperger's creates too much of a burden to get the details right," NJ.com reports. "There's also the danger that the other characters' insults about Sheldon's behavior—in other words, 90 percent of the show's comedy—would seem mean if they were mocking a medical condition as opposed to generic eccentricity. In general, it's more responsibility than they feel a relatively light comedy can handle."

Sorry, Sheldon is meant to be autistic.

The willingness to hoot and holler at a TV character perceived as different shows we may not be far from blackface. There was nothing particularly wrong with black people, they were just, well, funny, and it was funny to paint one's face and pretend.

No, it wasn't. And it's not now.

There's the equally important fact that Sheldon is an unreliable guide to what autism is really like. He's nothing like the mute, diapered, self-injurious kids who truly embody the epidemic or even the higher-functioning ones with no friends to show up at their birthday party.

Sheldon's is hardly the only autism portrayal in popular culture at the moment. As befits a rapidly growing phenomenon, autism is being picked up in books: *The Curious Incident of the Dog in the Nighttime*, which then became a Broadway hit with a Tony Award for its "autistic" lead; television programs—including *The A Word*, a six-episode series on Sundance in 2016—and a score of movies that either feature autism or showcase an autistic character in an important role. Feature film portrayals of autistic characters, of which there were less than a handful before the explosion of autism rates in 1988, have multiplied since Dustin Hoffman played Raymond Babbitt in *Rain Main*. A Wikipedia list of autistic characters in film currently counts sixty in the period from 1990 to 2016.

Many of these portrayals—starting with *Rain Man*—offer a much more realistic look at autism, although most abide by the bromides of mass entertainment: appealing and interesting characters work toward solutions that give viewers a sense that things get better when we all pull together. The publicity for *The A word* says that after the fictional family's five-year-old is diagnosed, they are shown "learning to deal with the diagnosis" and "facing differing parenting philosophies."

"[The show] is hopeful, honest and ultimately about the power of family and the range of issues that families can face together, from autism to aging to adultery," Joel Stillerman, president of original programming and development for AMC and SundanceTV, said in a press release. "We can't wait to share it with our growing universe of SundanceTV viewers."

The power of family, alas, is no defense against an autism diagnosis, and grouping it with aging and adultery as enduring facts of life is a strange ensemble.

More broadly, disability is being woven into entertainment in a way that goes a bit beyond inclusion and into immersion. In the movie *Finding Dory*, *every* main character is disabled in one way or the other, an upgrade, if you will, from its precursor *Finding Nemo*, in which the protagonist had one typical fin but most of the other characters were normally abled. In these Pixar fantasies, both Nemo and Dory manage to find their way home. Disability just takes a village to surmount. Then, of course, come the news segments, the televised benefits, and the documentaries that purport to show autistic people whose grit and special gifts lift them out of the pain of their disorder, at least long enough for grown men to cry and Jon Stewart to dab away a tear backstage (the mawkish beginning of *In a Different Key*).

This we have seen before, in the supposed triumph of Donald T. over autism due to the good-heartedness of his small-town Mississippi neighbors. We've seen it in the supposed return home of Asperger's "lost tribe." We've seen it in the autistic high school basketball player who goes on an inspirational three-point shooting spree. We've seen it in the supposedly "good news" stories of the store and school and Santa just for autistic children.

All this enables the Autism Epidemic to entangle itself in our sense of normality until the terrifying reality is replaced by a sense that things have always been this way and that it is somehow OK for them to continue.

◆ ◆ ◆

Along with becoming historicist—believing the trajectory of history is relentlessly upward—today's culture has become ahistorical, forgetting the recent past as soon as the calendar flips to a new year. Most autism "experts" don't want to look at the experience of real people like the frontline professionals who have observed the changes in the childhood population since the late 1980s. Yet, invariably when we talk to school nurses and others who see what's happening and have no reason to hide it, the idea that the rates are going up is axiomatic. They know that something's happening and there's nothing amusing or entertaining about it. What they see is a mounting toll of children and young adults who can't function in society. Pat Curtis worked for twenty-three years for the Oak Park-River Forest School District in suburban Chicago, evaluating elementary school kids who seemed to be struggling and assessing children as young as a few months before their third birthday.

"When I started in the district in 1986 there were a handful of children who had been identified as autistic—I mean single digits, maybe four or five. By the time I left in 2009 there were dozens and dozens," she said.

"It was very obvious to me that the numbers were rising. I would say that I probably sharpened my criteria, I was more aware of subtler symptoms of autism but in general my criteria did not change. I followed the guidelines because if they had four out of 7 characteristics I needed that to convince parents their child had autism." So much for the diagnosis shopping that Allen Frances said in chapter 6 was swelling the count of autistic children. Curtis counts one diagnosis-shopping family in twenty-three years! Other disorders have followed the same explosive upward trend, she said—ADHD, allergies, asthma.

◆ ◆ ◆

To us, the normalization of autism as a feel-good variation in human experience that creates "challenges" to meet and gifts like musical and math skills to compensate is pure kitsch. This is an urgent health crisis, a national emergency for which the correct response is not to be entertained but to be outraged. Yet, as we shared our ideas for this book with people we respect, we found not everyone agreed with our hard line on Sheldon Cooper.

"Actually I find *Big Bang Theory* quite funny," said one parent with two children on the spectrum. "I haven't seen every episode, but is Sheldon Cooper ever identified on camera as autistic, or did the Dark Side stick that label on him to serve their own nefarious purposes? But rather than attack the program (which would come off as sounding politically correct) you might say that yes, Sheldon is a funny eccentric physicist, but he bears no resemblance to typical autistic people, and we shouldn't get our ideas about autism from sitcoms."

A blog post[233] by Autism Speaks staffer Kerry Mugro, who has autism, writes: "Whether or not the Sheldon character has Asperger's, the show's popularity has brought this discussion to a large national audience, many of whom have high praise for Sheldon. I even heard this from a local boy with autism several weeks ago in a school that I visited. The boy wanted to grow up to be just like Sheldon! I have to admit that I have watched the show for years and I feel a connection to the character as well.

"Sheldon to me is one of the most unique characters we have on television today. As an aspiring consultant in the field of autism awareness and education, it's a message I want to impart to others. Even though Sheldon may seem different, a character like his should be treated with respect and tolerance. My message of respect and tolerance is one I hope organizations focus on. The wide spectrum of autism includes many truly unique individuals."

Sorry, we can't go along with that. The trouble is, injury does not deserve an amused live audience or even a laugh track. Far more often, autism is a tragedy for all involved, and both children and affected families are candid about it, though they often come from opposite ends of the spectrum of heartbreak. Here's an email Dan received at our blog from someone going by the pen name Potato Part.[234]

"I will preface this with the fact that I am autistic.

"I accidentally ran across Age of Autism. Age of Autism is the type of stuff that actually hurts autistic people. This type of thing makes it seem like the parents are suffering when their kids are autistic. That's complete bullshit.

"Those parents are the ones trying to kill us in an attempt to 'cure' us. It is definitely very nice to see that we are hated. I wanted to say thank you. Thank you for helping the content that hurts autistic people. Thank you for putting out content that gets autistic people killed. Thank you for actively harming autistic people. Thank you for reminding us that we are thought of as burdens.

"Thank you for making it harder for autistic people to live. Thank you for the content that makes autistic people suicidal. Thank you for making our life harder. Thank you for making our life worse."

A parent wrote us the following:[235]

"We have a 16 year old severe autistic child with violent behavior. We can't leave such a beautiful girl in this world alone after us. So we decided to live till we can bear. When we reach a point beyond which we can't pull any more, we will end our roles in this world along with her. People may call us escapists, but after taking this decision, we started enjoying life. We are sure nobody else can take care of such children other than parents.

"Doctors/scientists/bureaucrats/politicians—Put some more efforts/grant enough funds to research more to find solution ASAP to save families suffering from this problem."

Let's be clear here—the escape they're describing is murder-suicide.

Popularizing Sheldon is not going to make Potato Part feel more understood, and discussing parenting styles is not going to help this family. And even though murder and suicide are rare in autistic families, death in all its variety is never a remote prospect. Last year *Psychology Today* reported over one hundred known deaths of autistic children and adults have been attributed to wandering alone.[236]

◆ ◆ ◆

These numbers are set to increase. It is hard to believe, but with our recent spike in rates we are now just at the *beginning* of the Autism Epidemic. For many years, with US autism rates averaging around one in ten thousand, the total American autism population was very small. No one ever counted it, but in 1970, the total number of people with autism couldn't have been much higher than ten thousand. Since the turn of the hockey stick in 1988, autism populations have surged: first in children and recently in young adults. The Department of Education first started counting children with a school-based autism diagnosis in the 1995/6 school year. That count of children (not a perfect one, but the only data we have from a national registry of childhood disabilities) with an autism designation stood at twenty-eight thousand in 1995. By the 2013/4 school year, that number had soared to over half a million—autism surpassed intellectual disability for the first time in 2010—and shows no sign yet of leveling off. Even this surging number might be an underestimate: if you apply the autism rate of one in forty-five from a 2014 CDC survey measuring autism in children[237] (unlike the one in six-ty-eight rate from the CDC's ADDM Network, this survey probably had a fuller representation of children with Asperger's) to the entire United States, that gives us a current childhood population of over 1.6 million.

For the most part, American schools have absorbed the surge in the autistic childhood population quietly. Education in the United States, is an entitlement, and over the last couple of decades autism parents have won hard-fought access to educational services with local school boards (a story told well by Donvan and Zucker in *In a Different Key*). But serving over a million and a half special education students has been a wildly expensive proposition and local school budgets have strained to meet the demand. In Cambridge Massachusetts, where Mark has a child receiving special education services, fully 30 percent of the local school budget is devoted to providing special education services.

The story for adults is shaping up to be something quite different. As the first round of adults from the epidemic generation "age out" of the school system, the number of families with autistic young adults seeking services is just now becoming visible. As recently as 2010, the Social Security Administration started counting adults with autistic disorders for the first time. Like the childhood numbers in the mid-1990s, these counts started small—only seventy-two thousand in 2010. But in just five years that number has doubled, reflecting a growth rate of over 15 percent per year. If we project that rate forward for the next twenty-five years—a growth path that promises to take us to a one in forty-five rate of autistic adults by 2040—we can expect to see an

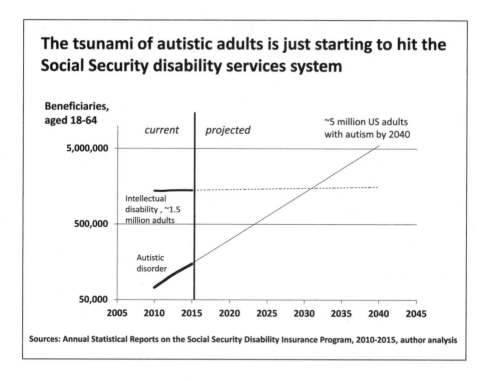

The tsunami of autistic adults is just starting to hit the Social Security disability services system

Beneficiaries, aged 18-64

current | *projected*

~5 million US adults with autism by 2040

5,000,000

Intellectual disability, ~1.5 million adults

500,000

Autistic disorder

50,000

2005 2010 2015 2020 2025 2030 2035 2040 2045

Sources: Annual Statistical Reports on the Social Security Disability Insurance Program, 2010-2015, author analysis

autistic population of over five million adults. That's an increase of thirty-three times over the current adult population.

The infrastructure to handle this surge in autistic adults—80 percent male, mostly young and physically strong, often violent, and with relatively little capacity for productive work—is nonexistent today. Further, the cost to serve this new population is entirely unbudgeted by the state-level disability service organizations that are tasked with providing them, and so will fall in large part to their parents, since disability services are not an entitlement and will almost certainly be curtailed as the unbudgeted demand for them rises.

Whoever bears them, the costs will be staggering.

One conservative estimate of the lifetime cost of a disabled person puts the number at $2 million. If we apply that number to a projected 2040 US population of autistic people of roughly 7 million (5 million adults plus about 2 million children), that yields a total lifetime cost of that new autistic population of around $14 trillion. Or, to put if differently, if we want to estimate the total *annual* cost of caring for that population, applying a conservative annual cost per autistic person of

$50,000 to that same population yields a run rate of $350 billion per year. In a world where the leading authorities are embracing Denier theories, we're not even remotely prepared to deal with cost increases of this magnitude.

◆ ◆ ◆

All this leaves autistic children, and their parents, without good alternatives. The following comment recently made the rounds of Facebook until it became converted to a meme.

"Every parent plans to raise their child for about 18 years, set them free for 30 years and then hope they come back to help them face the final years of their own life. A SPECIAL NEEDS parent plans to raise their child for 65 years and while doing so also has to prepare for the other 20 or so after they themselves are long gone. . . . Let that sink in for just a moment and you will begin to understand the drive and determination that many of us have while we are here on Earth."[238]

That scenario is a tragedy, not a sitcom.

◆ ◆ ◆

It's difficult to underestimate the dread, panic, and desperation with which parents of autistic children view the future. The American Dream of having a family and raising successful, independent children is getting smashed into pieces for the families affected by this new disorder. And since we have no experience as a society in which one in sixty-eight children grow into adulthood with autism, we are completely unprepared for what lies ahead: the escalating cost of services, the drain on caregivers, the frailty of elderly parents, the ripple effects on siblings and extended family, and the drag on the communities in which these exhausted families reside. The Denier impulse, to cheerfully whistle past the problem and declare it the next frontier of diversity awareness, is in no way a harmless theoretical stance. Rather, it is an abrogation of our civic responsibilities to one another. This injured autistic population is new. As we've said repeatedly, the rate of autism before 1930 was effectively zero. For a long time after it emerged, its frequency remained very low, but since the late 1980s the injury has

180

exploded. Its devastation lies all around us. And society is not prepared for how large it is going to become.

Autism parents often refer to a coming "tsunami" of autistic adults. The metaphor is apt. Like the new wave of autism, a tsunami drowns those families closest to the shoreline, but slowly and inexorably, its rising tide overwhelms human settlements far and wide, with a destructive power that makes them among the deadliest disasters known to man. Those of us who have been observing the autism epidemic for years have been trying our best to sound the tsunami warning. But the rising chorus of Denier propaganda threatens to drown us out before we can all recognize that the rising water level is not the coming of the high tide, but rather a disaster.

In an exquisite irony, autism (often parent) advocates are increasingly accused of being "anti-autism," of "ableism," and of intolerance toward this not-new, but simply neurodiverse population. To be sure, it is possible—indeed it is essential—to love and fully embrace the rights and promise of people, increasingly adults, with an autism diagnosis, while *at the same time* recognizing autism is a disability that can benefit from treatment—when the person themselves or their parent wishes it, to alleviate troubling symptoms and allow their true selves to emerge more fully. It is possible to love and respect the entire population of affected individuals *while at the same time* seeking to find the cause of an epidemic of environmental damage whose roots and rise must not be buried.

Love for a person with autism is a beautiful thing. Insanity in the form of Epidemic Denial is not. We cannot afford an unchecked autism epidemic. We must not accept the brutal injuries that have driven it. We have an obligation to end the epidemic and to put the Age of Autism in the rearview mirror. Epidemic Deniers need to come to their senses and get out of the way.

Notes

Prologue: Waiting

1. Arn van Krevelen, personal communication, January 7, 1963, in Bernard Rimland, *Infantile Autism: The Syndrome and Its Implications for a Neural Theory of Behavior* (Englewood Cliffs, N. J.: Prentice Hall, 1964).

Introduction: "What Hump?"

2. A recent survey (Benjamin Zablotsky et al., "Estimated Prevalence of Autism and Other Developmental Disabilities Following Questionnaire Changes in the 2014 National Health Interview Survey," *Natl Health Stat Report* 87 (2015): 1–20.) estimated U.S. autism prevalence in children aged 3–17 years old at 2.25%. Applied to a childhood population of 73 million, that rate places the US autism childhood population in 2014 at over 1.6 million. If one applies the CDC's latest reported autism rate of one in sixty-eight (or 1.47%) for children born in 2004 to the US childhood population (see Deborah L Christensen et al., "Prevalence and Characteristics of Autism Spectrum Disorder Among Children Aged 8 Years—Autism and Developmental Disabilities Monitoring Network, 11 Sites, United States, 2012," *MMWR Surveill Summ* 65 (3) (2016): 1–23), then the autism population is roughly 1.1 million.
3. A recent study estimated the lifetime costs of individuals with autism at between $1.4 million and $2.4 million (Ariane Beuscher et al., "Costs

of Autism Spectrum Disorders in the United Kingdom and the United States," *JAMA Pediatr* 168 (8) (2014): 721–8). An average lifetime cost of $2 million applied to a population of 1.1–1.6 million gives a total lifetime cost of the US childhood autism population of $2.2–3.2 trillion.

4. Mark Blaxill's testimony before the House Oversight and Government Reform Committee on the federal response to autism, "Mark Blaxill testifies before the Government Affairs Committee [sic] on Autism," https://www.youtube.com/watch?v=gy2ZcYqk4Bk.

5. Leo Kanner, "Autistic Disturbances of Affective Contact," *The Nervous Child* 2 (2) (1943): 217–250.

6. Steve Silberman, *NeuroTribes: The Legacy of Autism and the Future of Neurodiversity* (New York: Penguin, 2015).

7. "New Book Explores Autism from the First Case to Today," *ABC News*, http://abcnews.go.com/GMA/video/book-explores-autism-case -today-36355836.

8. Anne Bauer, " 'In a Different Key': A Cinematic, Sweeping Story of Autism," review of *In a Different Key: The Story of Autism*, by John Donvan and Caren Zucker, *The Washington Post*, January 29, 2015.

9. Stephen Moss, "Samuel Johnson Prize 2015," *The Guardian*, November 3, 2015.

10. "Autism Spectrum Disorder," *Centers for Disease Control and Prevention*, https://www.cdc.gov/ncbddd/autism/topics.html.

11. Todd Nelson, "Minnesota Autism Center School Plans Expansion in Eagan," *The Star-Tribune*, April 14, 2015.

12. Hosea Sanders, "Toy Store for Children on Autism Spectrum Opens in Chicago," *ABC Eyewitness News (WLS)*, November 13, 2016, http:// abc7chicago.com/family/toy-store-for-children-on-autism-spectrum-opens-in-chicago/1604040/.

13. H. L. Doherty, "Autism Expert Paul Offit and Neurodiversity Ideology," *Facing Autism in New Brunswick*, February 1, 2011, http://autisminnb. blogspot.com/2011/02/autism-expert-paul-offit-and.html.

14. Silberman, *NeuroTribes*, 469–70.

15. J. B. Handley, "Paul Offit and the 'Original Sin' of Autism," *Age of Autism*, January 31, 2011, http://www.ageofautism.com/2011/01/paul-offit-and-the-original-sin-of-autism.html.

16. "UC Davis M.I.N.D. Institute Study Shows California's Autism Increase Not Due to Better Counting, Diagnosis," *U.C. Davis Health*

System, February 19, 2009, http://www.ucdmc.ucdavis.edu/welcome/features/20090218_autism_environment/.

17. "Federal Response to Rise in Autism Rates," *C-SPAN 3*, November 29, 2012, https://www.c-span.org/video/?309672–1/federal-response-rise-autism-rates/.

18. Bauer, review of *Different Key*.

19. John Donvan and Caren Zucker, *In a Different Key: The Story of Autism* (New York: Crown Publishers, 2016), 432.

20. Donvan and Zucker, *Different Key*, xi.

21. Katie Wright, "NIH Autism Regression Study Attempts to Ferret out Answers," *Age of Autism*, March 10, 2016, http://www.ageofautism.com/2016/03/nih-autism-regression-study-attempts-to-ferret-out-answers.html.

22. Bernard Rimland, personal communication to Mark Blaxill, April 18, 2003.

23. Donvan and Zucker, *Different Key*, 433.

Chapter 1: Desperately Seeking Gulliver

24. Wilhelm Weygandt, "Idiotie und Dementia Praecox," *Zeitschrift flir die Erforschun und Behandlung des jugendlichen Schwachsinns* I (1907): 3II.

25. Weygandt, "Idiotie und Dementia Praecox."

26. Leo Kanner, undated item, Kanner archive at the American Psychiatric Association; Kanner appears to have garbled Weygandt's account, which as we will see included just one child with early-onset symptoms Kanner may have been comparing to autism.

27. Eugen Bleuler, *Dementia Praecox: Or the Group of Schizophrenias* (New York: International Universities Press, 1911).

28. Theodor Heller, "Uber Dementia infantilis," *Zeitschrift fur Kinderforschung* 37 (1930): 661–667. Autistic children for the most part were, like Weygandt's case, profoundly disabled,

29. Alexander Westphal et al., "Revisiting Regression in Autism: Heller's Dementia Infantilis, (Includes a translation of 'Über Dementia Infantilis')," *J Autism Dev Disord* 43 (2) (2013): 265–71, citing Theodor Heller, "Uber Dementia infantilis: Verblodungsprozen im Kindesalter," *Zeitschrift fur die Erforschung und Behandlung des Jugendlichen Schwachsinns* 2 (1908): 17–28.

Chapter 2: Absence of Evidence: Gulliver in Lilliput

30. Samuel Gridley Howe, *Report Made to the Legislature of Massachusetts, Upon Idiocy* (Boston: Coolidge & Wiley, 1848).
31. John Langdon Down, "On Some of the Mental Affections of Childhood and Youth," *Lettsomian Lectures* (London: J & A Churchill, 1887).
32. William Wotherspoon Ireland, *The Mental Affections of Children: Idiocy, Imbecility and Insanity* (London: J. & A. Churchill, 1898).
33. Alfred Frank Tredgold, *Mental Deficiency: Amentia* (New York: William Wood and Company: 1920).
34. Tredgold, *Mental Deficiency: Amentia*, 319.
35. Tredgold, *Mental Deficiency: Amentia*, 320–1.
36. Kanner, "Autistic Disturbances."
37. Ireland, *Mental Affections*.
38. Ireland, *Mental Affections*, 271–302.
39. Ireland, *Mental Affections*, vii–ix.
40. J. Langdon H. Down, "Observations on an Ethnic Classification of Idiots," *London Hospital Reports* 3 (1886): 259–62.
41. Darrell A. Treffert, "Dr. J. Langdon Down and Developmental Disorders," 2004, retrieved September 2, 2005, from *Wisconsin Medical Society*, www.wisconsinmedicalsociety.org/savant_syndrome/savant_articles/doctor_down.
42. John Donvan and Caren Zucker, "The Early History of Autism in America," *Smithsonian Magazine*, January 2016.
43. When one of us was a reporter, it was common in journalism to refer to the "to be sure" paragraph, a hedge on criticism that alternative explanations were not considered; most such "to be sure" paragraphs are not quite so self-negating.
44. Jonathan Rose, "Yes, There Is an Autism Epidemic," *History News Network*, March 6, 2016, http://historynewsnetwork.org/article/161992.
45. Rose, "Autism Epidemic."
46. Howe, *Upon Idiocy*, 10–11.
47. Howe, *Upon Idiocy*, 10–11.
48. Rose, "Autism Epidemic."
49. John Haslam, *Observations on Madness and Melancholy* (London: G. Hayden, 1809).
50. Jean-Etienne Esquirol, *Mental Maladies: A Treatise on Insanity* (Philadelphia: Lea and Blanchard, 1845).

51. Henry Maudsley, *The Physiology and Pathology of the Mind* (New York: D. Appleton & Company, 1867).

52. Haslam, *Madness and Melancholy*, 185–7.

53. Haslam, *Madness and Melancholy*, 188–91.

54. Esquirol, *Mental Maladies*, 33.

55. Esquirol, *Mental Maladies*, 34.

56. Leo Kanner, "Childhood Psychosis: A Historical Overview," *J Autism Child Schizophr* 1 (1) (1971): 14–9.

57. Eli A. Rubinstein, "Childhood Mental Disease in America: A Review of the Literature before 1900," *American Journal of Orthopsychiatry* 18 (2) (1948): 314–32.

58. Rubinstein, "Childhood Mental Disease in America."

59. Maudsley, *Physiology and Pathology*, 259–93.

60. Maudsley, *Physiology and Pathology*, 259–93.

61. Michael Macdonald, *Mystical Bedlam: Madness, Anxiety, and Healing in Seventeenth-Century England* (Cambridge: Cambridge University Press, 1981), 31.

62. M. Waltz and P. Shattock, "Autistic Disorder in Nineteenth-Century London: Three Case Reports," *Autism* 8 (1) (2004): 7–20.

Chapter 3: Evidence of Absence: The Empty Quadrant

63. Irving Marmer Copi, *Introduction to Logic* (New York: Macmillan, 1953), 95.

64. Melissa Dahl, "A Leading Autism Organization Is No Longer Searching for a "Cure,"" *New York*, October 18, 2016.

65. Steve Silberman, "The Geek Syndrome," *Wired*, December 1, 2001.

66. Kanner, "Autistic Disturbances of Affective Contact."

67. Leo Kanner, "Early Infantile Autism," *J Pediatr* 25 (3) (1944): 211–217.

68. Leon Eisenberg and Leo Kanner, "Childhood Schizophrenia; Symposium, 1955. VI. Early Infantile Autism 1943–55," *Am J Orthopsychiatry* 26 (3) (1956): 556–66.

69. Michael Rutter, "Diagnosis and Definition," in *Autism: a Reappraisal of Concepts and Treatments*, Michael Rutter and Eric Schopler, editors (New York: Plenum Press, 1978).

70. Rutter, "Diagnosis and Definition," 19.

71. Rutter, "Diagnosis and Definition," 7.

72. Leo Kanner, "In Defense of the Parent," *The New York Times Magazine*, February 4, 1940, 100.

73. Donvan and Zucker, *Different Key*, 41.

74. E. Shorter and L. E. Wachtel, "Childhood Catatonia, Autism and Psychosis past and Present: Is There an 'Iron Triangle'?" *Acta Psychiatr Scand* 128 (1) (2013): 21–33.

75. Leo Kanner, *Child Psychiatry* (Baltimore: Charles C. Thomas, 1935).

76. Leo Kanner, *Child Psychiatry: Third Edition* (Springfield: Charles C. Thomas, 1967).

77. Bernard Rimland, *Infantile Autism: The Syndrome and Its Implications for a Neural Theory of Behavior* (Englewood Cliffs, NJ: Prentice Hall, 1964).

78. Kanner L, Rodriguez A, Ashenden B. "How Far Can Autistic Children Go in Matters of Social Adaptation?" *J Autism Child Schizophr* 2 (1) (1972): 9–33.

79. Yakovlev, P. I., Weinburger, M., and Chipman, C. C. "Heller's Syndrome as a Pattern of Schizophrenic Behavior Disorder in Early Childhood," *Am J Ment Deficiency* 53 (1948): 318–33, 7.

80. Lauretta Bender, "Childhood Schizophrenia: Clinical Study of One Hundred Schizophrenic Children," *American Journal of Orthopsychiatry* 17 (1) (1947): 40–56.

81. G. E. Sukharava, "Die schizoiden Psychopathien im Kindesalter," translated by Sula Wolff, *Monatsschrift für Psychiatrie und Neurologie*, 1926.

82. Lightner Witmer, "Orthogenic Cases, XIV—Don: A Curable Case of Arrested Development Due to a Fear Psychosis the Result of Shock in a Three Year Old Infant [sic]," *Psychol Clinic* 13 (1919–22): 97–111.

83. Rimland, *Infantile Autism*, 6.

84. Witmer, "Orthogenic Cases."

85. L. A. Lurie and S. Levy, "Personality Changes and Behavior Disorders of Children Following Pertussis: A Report Based on the Study of Five Hundred Problem Children," *JAMA* 120 (12) (1942): 890–894.

86. C. L. Davidson and Jean Terry Thomas, "Post-Vaccinial Encephalitis," *Archives of Disease in Childhood* 17 (1942): 162.

87. George C. Darr and Frederic G. Worden, "Case Report Twenty-Eight Years After an Infantile Autistic Disorder," *The American Journal of Orthopsychiatry* 21 (3) (1951): 559–70.

88. Darr and Worden, "Case Report Twenty-Eight Years After an Infantile Autistic Disorder."

89. Jakob Lutz, "Uber die Schizophrenie im Kindesalter," *Schweiz Archiv Neurol Psychiatr* 39 (1937): 335–372 and 40: 141–163. Translated by Birgit Calhoun.

90. Herbert Jancke, "Zwei Faile von Dementia infantilis," *Arch. f. Kinderh* 88 (1929): 114–127. Translated by Birgit Calhoun.

91. Hans Asperger, "'Autistic Psychopathy' in Childhood," 1944, edited, translated, and annotated by Uta Frith in *Autism and Asperger Syndrome* (Cambridge: Cambridge University Press, 1991), 37–92.

92. N. Moritz Tramer, "Tagebuch über ein geistekrankes Kind.," *Ztschr f Kinderpsychiat* (1934–5): 91 et seq. Translated by Birgit Calhoun.

93. Akira Hashimoto, "A 'German World' Shared Among Doctors: A History of the Relationship Between Japanese and German Psychiatry before World War II," *Hist Psychiatry* 24 (2) (2013): 180–95.

Chapter 4: Autism Arrives

94. Hans Asperger, "Das Psychisch Abnormale Kind," *Wiener Klinische Wochenschrift* 51 (1938): 1314–1317. Translated by Birgit Calhoun.

95. "First Ladies: Harriet Lane," The White House, https://www.white-house.gov/1600/first-ladies/harrietlane.

96. Kanner, "Autistic Disturbances."

97. Leo Kanner, letter to Ernest Harms, January 19, 1942, in American Psychological Association archives.

98. Silberman, *NeuroTribes*, 171.

99. Silberman, *NeuroTribes*, 168.

100. Silberman, *NeuroTribes*, 168.

101. Kanner, "Autistic Disturbances."

102. Silberman, *NeuroTribes*, 176.

103. Silberman, *NeuroTribes*, 221–2.

104. Georg Frankl, "Language and Affective Contact," *Nervous Child* 2 (3) (1943): 251–262.

105. Georg Frankl, "Autism in Childhood: An Attempt of an Analysis (unpublished manuscript)," Lawrence, KS: Kenneth Spencer Research Library, The University of Kansas (1957).

106. John Elder Robison, "Kanner, Asperger, and Frankl: A Third Man at the Genesis of the Autism Diagnosis," *Autism*, September 13, 2016 [Epub ahead of print].

107. Silberman, *NeuroTribes*, 216.
108. Donvan and Zucker, *Different Key*, 35.
109. Donvan and Zucker, *Different Key*, 36–7.
110. Simon Baron-Cohen, "Did Hans Asperger Save Children from the Nazis—or Sell Them Out?" *The Spectator*, September 12, 2015.
111. Donvan and Zucker, *Different Key*, 566–7.
112. Grunya E Sukhareva, "Die schizoiden Psychopathien im Kindesalter," translated by Sula Wolff, *Monatsschrift für Psychiatrie und Neurologie*, 1926.
113. Anni B. Weiss, "Qualitative Intelligence Testing as a Means of Diagnosis in the Examination of Psychopathic Children," *American Journal of Orthopsychiatry* 5 (2) (1935): 154–179.
114. Asperger, "Das Psychisch Abnormale Kind."
115. Hans Asperger, "Die 'Autistischen Psychopathen' im Kindesalter," *Archiv für Psychiatrie und Nervenkrankheiten* 117(1) (1944): 76–136. Translated by Birgit Calhoun.
116. D. Arn van Krevelen, "Early Infantile Autism and Autistic Psychopathy," *J Autism Child Schizophr* 1(1) (1971): 82–6.
117. Wolfgang Brezinska, *"Orthopedagogy at the Faculty of Medicine at the University of Vienna: Its story from 1911–1985,"* *Zeitschrift für Pädagogik* 43 (2) (1997): 395–420. Translated by Birgit Calhoun.
118. Joseph J Michaels, "The Heilpedagogical Station of the Children's Clinic at the University of Vienna," *American Journal of Orthopsychiatry* 5 (3) (1935): 266–275.
119. Georg Frankl, "Ordering and obeying," *Zeitschrift fur Kinderforschung* 42 (1933): 464.
120. Asperger, "Das Psychisch Abnormale Kind."
121. Donvan and Zucker, *Different Key*, 335.
122. Adam Feinstein, *A History of Autism: Conversations with the Pioneers* (West Sussex: Wiley-Blackwell, 2010), 17.
123. John Donvan and Caren Zucker, "The Doctor and the Nazis," *Tablet*, January 19, 2016. http://www.tabletmag.com/jewish-life-and-religion/196348/the-doctor-and-the-nazis.
124. Franz Hamburger, *Die Neurosen des Kindesalters* (Stuttgart: Ferdinand Enke Verlag, 1939).
125. Kathrin Hippler and Christian Klicpera, "A Retrospective Analysis of the Clinical Case Records of 'Autistic Psychopaths' Diagnosed by Hans

Asperger and His Team at the University Children's Hospital, Vienna," *Philos Trans R Soc Lond B Biol Sci* 358 (1430) (2003): 291–301.

Chapter 5: Unqualified Observers

126. Leo Kanner, "Citation Classic—Autistic Disturbances of Affective Contact," *Current Contents* 25 (1979): 14.
127. Dan Olmsted, "The Age of Autism: Case 1 Revisited," *United Press International*, August 15, 2005, http://www.upi.com/Health_News/2005/08 /15/The-Age-of-Autism-Case-1-revisited/UPI-96511124113501/.
128. Leon Eisenberg, "The Autistic Child in Adolescence," *The American Journal of Psychiatry* 112 (1956): 607–12.
129. "Histoire, Histoires D'Autisme," Anne Georget, Gloria Films, 2000.
130. Erica Gunderson, "New Book 'In a Different Key' Tells the History, Politics of Autism," *Chicago Tonight, WTTW*, February 8, 2016, http: //chicagotonight.wttw.com/2016/02/08/new-book-different-key -tells-history-politics-autism.
131. Gunderson, "New Book."
132. Jennie Rothenberg Gritz, "Finding Donald," *The Atlantic*, September 14, 2010, https://www.theatlantic.com/video/index/62806/finding-donald/.
133. Personal communication from John Donvan to Dan Olmsted, January 4, 2017.
134. "Autism's First Child," *Good Morning America, ABC News*, September 15, 2010, http://abcnews.go.com/GMA/autisms-child-donald-gray-triplett -person-diagnosed/story?id=11632605.
135. "A Personal Journey Covering Autism 'In a Different Key,'" *ABC News Nightline*, January 20, 2016, http://abcnews.go.com/Nightline/video/ personal-journey-covering-autism-key-36391088.
136. George Stephanopoulos, "New Book Explores Autism from the First Case to Today," *Good Morning America*, January 18, 2016, http://abcnews. go.com/GMA/video/book-explores-autism-case-today-36355836.
137. Stephanopoulos, "New Book."
138. Donvan and Zucker, *Different Key*, 568.
139. "Mother Helped Break Down Barriers for Children with Autism," *ABC News Nightline*, January 15, 2016.
140. Dan Olmsted and Mark Blaxill, *The Age of Autism: Mercury, Medicine and a Man-made Epidemic* (New York: Thomas Dunne, 2010), 24–30.

141. Silberman, *NeuroTribes*, 150.

142. Silberman, *NeuroTribes*, 19–32.

143. George Wilson, *The Life of the Hon. Henry Cavendish,* (London: Cavendish Society, 1851), 167.

144. Henry Cavendish, "Observations on Mr. Hutchins's Experiments for Determining the Degree of Cold at Which Quicksilver Freezes," *Phil Trans R So Lond* 73(1) (1783): 303–328.

145. Wilson, *Hon. Henry Cavendish.*

146. H. A. Waldron, "Did the Mad Hatter Have Mercury Poisoning?" *Br Med J (Clin Res Ed)* 287 (6409) (1983): 1961.

147. Silberman, *NeuroTribes*, 419.

148. "Notice to Readers: Thimerosal in Vaccines: A Joint Statement of the American Academy of Pediatrics and the Public Health Service," *MMWR*, 48 (26) (1999): 563–565.

149. David Kirby, *Evidence of Harm: Mercury in Vaccines and the Autism Epidemic: A Medical Controversy* (New York: St. Martin's Press, 2005), 172.

150. Donvan and Zucker, *Different Key*, 479.

151. Kirby, *Evidence of Harm*, 253.

152. Donvan and Zucker, *Different Key*, 440.

153. Personal communication from Andrew Wakefield to Dan Olmsted, date unknown.

154. John Donvan and Caren Zucker, "Five Tips for Candidates Who Want to Talk about Autism—Responsibly," *The Washington Post*, February 11, 2016, https://www.washingtonpost.com/opinions/here-is-the-conversation -candidates-should-be-having-about-autism/2016/02/11/19d208b0 -cb49–11e5-a7b2–5a2f824b02c9_story.html?utm_term=.963c2b728d70.

155. Van Krevelen, "Early Infantile Autism and Autistic Psychopathy."

156. D. Arn van Krevelen, "Early Infantile Autism," *Z. f. Kinderpsychiat* 19 (1952): 91–7, cited in Rimland, "Infantile Autism."

157. Louise Despert to Leo Kanner, July 12, 1943, letter, APA archives.

158. Leo Kanner to Louise Despert, July 15, 1943, letter, APA archives.

159. Leo Kanner to Louise Despert, November 1944 letter, APA archives.

160. Howard Potter, "Schizophrenia in children," *Am J Psychiatry* 89 (1933): 1253–1270.

161. Mildred Creak, "Psychoses in Children," *Proc Roy Soc Med* 31 (1938): 519–28.

162. E. Grebelskaya-Albatz, "Zur Klinik der Schizophrenien des frühen Kindesalters," *Schweiz Arch Neurol Psychia* 34 (1934): 244. Also, E. Grebelskaya-Albatz, "Zur Klinik der Schizophrenien des frühen Kindesalters," *Schweiz Arch Neurol Psychiat* 35 (1935): 30.

163. J. Franklin Robinson and Louis J. Vitale, "Children with circumscribed interest patterns," *Am J Orthopsychiatry* 24 (4) (1954): 755–66.

164. Van Krevelen, "Early Infantile Autism and Autistic Psychopathy."

165. D. Arn van Krevelen and Christine Kuipers, "The Psychopathology of Autistic Psychopathy," *Acta Paedopsychiatr* 29 (1962): 22–31.

166. "Hopkins Doctor Tells of Maryland Boy, 4, Who 'Read' English and German," undated newspaper article, Johns Hopkins archives.

Chapter 6: The Epidemic and Its Implications

167. Del Bigtree at the Real Truth About Health Conference, Orlando Florida, September 10, 2016.

168. Allen Frances, *Saving Normal: An Insider's Revolt Against Out-of-Control Psychiatric Diagnosis, DSM-5, Big Pharma, and the Medicalization of Ordinary Life*, (New York: William Morrow, 1994).

169. Deborah L Christensen et al., "Prevalence and Characteristics of Autism Spectrum Disorder Among Children Aged 8 Years—Autism and Developmental Disabilities Monitoring Network, 11 Sites, United States, 2012," *MMWR Surveill Summ* 65 (3) (2016): 1–23.

170. California Department of Developmental Services, "Changes in the Population of Persons with Autism and Pervasive Developmental Disorders in California's Developmental Services System: 1987 through 1998," A Report to the Legislature, Department of Developmental Services, Sacramento, California (1999).

171. Fred R. Volkmar, Ami Klin, and D. J. Cohen, "Diagnosis and Classification of Autism and Related Conditions: Consensus and Issues," in *Handbook of Autism and Pervasive Developmental Disorders, 2nd ed.*, D. J. Cohen and F. R. Volkmar, editors (New York: John Wiley and Sons, 1997), 5–40.

172. "Autism expert Paul Offit and Neurodiversity ideology" February 1, 2011, http://autisminnb.blogspot.com/2011/02/autism-expert-paul-offit-and.html.

173. E. Fuller Torrey, Stephen P. Hersh, and Kinne D. McCabe, "Early Childhood Psychosis and Bleeding during Pregnancy—A Prospective Study of Gravid Women and Their Offspring," *Journal of Autism and Childhood Schizophrenia* 5 (4) (1975): 287–97.

174. See T. S. Brugha et al., "The Proportion of True Cases of Autism is Not Changing, *BMJ* 348 (2014), and T. S. Brugha et al., "Autistic Spectrum Disorders in Adults Living in Households Throughout England: Report from the Adult Psychiatric Morbidity Survey 2007," *U.K. National Health Service*, September 22, 2009, http://content.digital.nhs.uk/pubs/asdpsychiatricmorbidity07.

175. John Stone, "Not Allowed on Pubmed Commons: Reply to Prof Brugha on the UK Adult Autism Survey," *Age of Autism*, September 26, 2016, http://www.ageofautism.com/2016/09/not-allowed-on-pubmed-commons-reply-to-prof-brugha-on-the-uk-adult-autism-survey.html.

176. Olmsted and Blaxill, *Age of Autism*, 234.

177. California Department of Developmental Services, "Changes in the Population of Persons with Autism and Pervasive Developmental Disorders in California's Developmental Services System: 1987 through 1998."

178. Lisa A. Croen et al., "The Changing Prevalence of Autism in California," *Journal of Autism and Developmental Disorders* 32 (2002): 207–15.

179. Eric Fombonne, Editorial Commentary, *Journal of Autism and Developmental Disorders* 32 (3) (2002): 151– 52.

180. Mark F. Blaxill, David S. Baskin, and Walter O. Spitzer, "Commentary: Blaxill, Baskin, and Spitzer on Croen et al. (2002), 'The Changing Prevalence of Autism in California,'" *Journal of Autism and Developmental Disorders* 33 (2) (2003).

181. R. S. Byrd et al., "Report to the Legislature on the Principal Findings from the Epidemiology of Autism in California: A Comprehensive Pilot Study," *Davis (CA): MIND Institute*, October 17, 2002.

182. Lisa A. Croen and Judith K. Grether, "Response: A Response to 'Blaxill, Baskin, and Spitzer on Croen et al. (2002), "The Changing Prevalence of Autism in California,"'" *Journal of Autism and Developmental Disorders* 33 (2003): 227–9.

183. California Department of Developmental Services, "Autistic Spectrum Disorders: Changes in the California Caseload, an Update: 1999 through 2002," Sacramento: California Health and Human Services Agency, Department of Developmental Services, 2003.

184. J. G. Gurney et al., "Analysis of Prevalence Trends of Autism Spectrum Disorder in Minnesota," *Arch Pediatr Adolesc Med* 157 (2003): 622–7.
185. C. J. Newschaffer, M. D. Falb, and J. G. Gurney, "National Autism Prevalence Trends from United States Special Education Data," *Pediatrics* 115 (3) (2005): e277–82.
186. Centers for Disease Control and Prevention, "Prevalence of Autism Spectrum Disorders—Autism and Developmental Disabilities Monitoring Network, Six Sites, United States, 2000," *MMWR* 56 (No. SS-1) (2007).
187. Marshalyn Yeargin-Allsopp et al., "Prevalence of Autism in a US Metropolitan Area," *JAMA*, 289 (1) (2003): 49–55.
188. Kim Van Naarden Braun et al., "Trends in the Prevalence of Autism Spectrum Disorder, Cerebral Palsy, Hearing loss, Intellectual Disability, and Vision Impairment, Metropolitan Atlanta, 1991–2010," *PLoS One* 10 (4) (2015): e0124120.
189. Paul T. Shattuck, "The contribution of Diagnostic Substitution to the Growing Administrative Prevalence of Autism in US Special Education," *Pediatrics* 117 (4) (2006):1028–37.
190. Donvan and Zucker, *Different Key*, 423.
191. Donvan and Zucker, *Different Key*, p 427
192. "Jerry Seinfeld to Brian Williams: 'I think I'm on the Spectrum," *NBC Nightly News*, November 6, 2014, http://www.nbcnews.com/nightly-news/jerry-seinfeld-brian-williams-i-think-im-spectrum-n242941.
193. "Jerry Seinfeld Clarifies Autism Comments, Decides He's Not on the Spectrum After All," *US Weekly*, November 21, 2014.
194. Richard Roy Grinker, *Unstrange Minds: Remapping the World of Autism* (New York: Basic Books, 2007).
195. Claudia Wallis, "Is the Autism Epidemic a Myth?" *TIME*, January 12, 2007.
196. Silberman, *NeuroTribes*, 401.

Chapter 7: The Dynamics of Denial

197. Karl Raimund Popper, *The Poverty of Historicism* (London: Routledge and Kegan Paul, 1974 reprint) 88–9.
198. "Jenny McCarthy and Jim Carrey Discuss Autism; Medical Experts Weigh In," *Larry King Live: CNN*, April 3, 2009, http://transcripts.cnn.com/transcripts/0904/03/lkl.01.html.

199. W. H. Auden, "The Unknown Citizen," from *Another Time* (New York: Random House, 1940).

200. *Manville Personal Injury Settlement Trust*, https://mantrust.claimsres.com/.

201. "Dan Olmsted," *Wikipedia*, https://en.wikipedia.org/wiki/Dan_Olmsted.

202. "Toxic Chemicals," *National Resources Defense Council*, https://www.nrdc.org/issues/toxic-chemicals.

203. Gardiner Harris and Anahad O'Connor, "On Autism's Cause, It's Parents Versus Research," *The New York Times*, June 25, 2005.

204. Philip J. Landrigan. "What Causes Autism? Exploring the Environmental Contribution," *Curr Opin Pediatr* 22 (2) (2010): 219–25.

205. Cynthia D. Nevison, "A Comparison of Temporal Trends in United States Autism Prevalence to Trends in Suspected Environmental Factors," *Environ Health* 13 (2014): 73.

206. "Encyclopedia of American Loons," http://americanloons.blogspot.com/.

207. Jamie Wells, "Debunking Vaccine Myths with Dr. Paul Offit," *American Council on Science and Health*, October 7, 2016, http://www.acsh.org/news/2016/10/07/debunking-vaccine-myths-dr-paul-offit-10269.

208. Hank Campbell, "3 Reasons Aerial Pesticides Are Not Causing Autism," *American Council on Science and Health*, May 2, 2016, http://acsh.org/news/2016/05/02/3-reasons-aerial-pesticides-are-not-causing-autism.

209. Andy Kroll and Jeremy Schulman, "Leaked Documents Reveal the Secret Finances of a Pro-Industry Science Group," *Mother Jones*, October 28, 2013.

210. "Estimates of Funding for Various Research, Condition, and Disease Categories (RCDC)," *NIH*, February 10, 2016, https://report.nih.gov/categorical_spending.aspx.

211. Mark Blaxill and Dan Olmsted, "A License to Kill?" in *Vaccine Epidemic: How Corporate Greed, Biased Science, and Coercive Government Threaten Our Human Rights, Our Health, and Our Children*, Mary Holland and Louise Habakus, editors (New York: Skyhorse Publishing, 2011).

212. Author analysis of public financial statements of named companies.

213. There were 28,660 pediatricians in the United States in 2015. Their average take-home pay is $183,000 (https://www.bls.gov/oes/current/oes291065.htm). Their typical practice takes in more like $666K per pediatrician year on average (see "2016 Physician Inpatient/Outpatient Revenue Survey," *Merritt Hawkins* https://www.merritthawkins.com/uploadedFiles/MerrittHawkins/Surveys/

Merritt_Hawkins-2016_RevSurvey.pdf). That suggests that the industry size for the United States only is around $19 billion.

214. "Medicines in Development: Vaccines—A Report on the Prevention and Treatment of Disease through Vaccines," *America's Biopharmaceutical Research Companies*, 2013 Report, http://phrma.org/sites/default/files/pdf/Vaccines_2013.pdf.

215. Author Stephen King tweet, November 9, 2015, https://twitter.com/stephenking/status/663768619692724224?lang=en.

216. Mark Blaxill, "Offit Cashes In: Closing the Books on the Vaccine Profits of a Merck-Made Millionaire," *Age of Autism,* January 31, 2011, http://www.ageofautism.com/2011/01/offit-cashes-in-closing-the-books-on-the-vaccine-profits-of-a-merck-made-millionaire-1.html.

217. "AMA Calls for Ban on DTC Ads of Prescription Drugs and Medical Devices," *American Medical Association*, November 17, 2015, https://www.ama-assn.org/content/ama-calls-ban-direct-consumer-advertising-prescription-drugs-and-medical-devices.

218. Jesse Ventura, "Robert F. Kennedy Jr. Takes on Big Pharma & the Vaccine Industry," *Off the Grid*, May 18, 2015, http://www.ora.tv/offthegrid/2015/5/18/grid-robert—kennedy-jr-takes-big-pharma—vaccine-industry-0_6ck7ne6j25bv.

219. Personal communication to authors from Sharyl Attkisson, date unknown.

220. Dan Schulman, "Drug Test," *The Columbia Journalism Review*, November/December 2005.

221. Curtis Brainard, "Sticking with the Truth: How 'Balanced' Coverage Helped Sustain the Bogus Claim that Childhood Vaccines Can Cause Autism," *The Columbia Journalism Review*, May/June 2013.

222. Popper, *Poverty of Historicism*.

223. Harris and O'Connor, "Parents Versus Research."

224. "Statement from William Thompson Re *Pediatrics* MMR African American Males Data," *Age of Autism*, August 27, 2004, http://www.ageofautism.com/2014/08/statement-from-william-thompson-re-pediatrics-mmr-african-american-males-data.html.

225. "Robert De Niro Debates Autism's Link to Vaccines on TODAY Show," *The Today Show*, April 15, 2016, http://www.today.com/popculture/robert-deniro-debates-autism-s-link-vaccines-today-show-t86136.

226. Bobbie Gallagher, *A Brick Wall: How a Boy with No Words Spoke to the World* (Charleston: CreateSpace, 2016), 66–9.

227. Gallagher, *Brick Wall*.

228. Joseph Mercola, "Bush Plans to Veto Removal of Mercury from Infant Vaccines," *Organic Consumers Association*, July 24, 2007, https://www.organicconsumers.org/news/bush-plans-veto-removal-mercury-infant-vaccines.

229. Texas State Attorney Nico Lahood interview, "Vaxxed Stories: The Prosecutor," August 30, 2016, https://www.youtube.com/watch?v=Pi9PNKW7w3Q.

230. "Our Principles," *The Canary Party*, http://canaryparty.org/principles/.

Epilogue: Normalizing Autism

231. Tony Maglio, "'Big Bang Theory': How Its Ratings Are Different Than Every Other Show," *The Wrap*, May 4, 2016, http://www.thewrap.com/big-bang-theory-tv-ratings-season-9-finale-cbs/.

232. Alan Sepinwall, "Does Sheldon from 'Big Bang Theory' have Asperger's?" *NJ.com*, August 13, 2009, http://www.nj.com/entertainment/tv/index.ssf/2009/08/reader_mail_does_sheldon_from.html.

233. Kerry Mugro, "Why Our Autism Community Loves Sheldon Cooper," *Autism Speaks*, August 13, 2014, https://www.autismspeaks.org/blog/2014/08/13/why-our-autism-community-loves-sheldon-cooper.

234. Dan Olmsted, "Don't Be Cruel," *Age of Autism,* September 17, 2016, http://www.ageofautism.com/2016/09/age-of-autism-weekly-wrap-dont-be-cruel.html.

235. Olmsted, "Don't Be Cruel."

236. Amy S. F. Lutz, "117 Autistic Children and Adults Who Died Deserve Better," *Psychology Today*, December 20, 2016.

237. Zablotsky, "Estimated Prevalence."

238. Dale Jackson, Facebook post, March 13, 2016.

Acknowledgments

This book reflects the collective insights and efforts of many people. It is a pleasure to thank them here.

Our first debt is to Birgit Calhoun, whose translations of numerous German medical journal articles—some never before in English—deepened our understanding of childhood mental illness and the milieu in which autism was first observed. The citations we found in one paper often led us to dig up another, but Birgit was always available for another round of reading and discussion. A German native who huddled in subways during World War II air raids, she was an invaluable member of our team.

We appreciate the input from a wide range of early readers, including Jonathan Rose, Brooke Potthast, Rosamond McDonel, Jennifer Larson, Dan Burns, Mark Milett, John Stone, Kim Stagliano, and Teresa Conrick; the Age of Autism community online; and the families that have generously shared their stories with us.

Our book dedication to the late Bernard Rimland reflects his impact not just on thousands of people with autism but on both of us. Dan met "Bernie" at a breakfast in Virginia during an autism conference. He asked Dan to colead a discussion with him that turned out to be his last public appearance. Dan feels Bernie lightly "tapped" him to continue a journalistic approach to the autism epidemic, and he considers it both an honor and an obligation to do so. Mark was encouraged by Bernie to use his wide knowledge base and expert analytical background to take down the Epidemic Denial argument.

And so in this, our third book together, we salute Bernie and his commitment to find the truth and help sick kids. We hope our work contributes to those goals.

Coauthor's note

Dan Olmsted passed away unexpectedly on January 20, 2017, shortly after we submitted the final manuscript of *Denial*. Dan was a pioneering investigative journalist, a gifted writer, and a breathtakingly original thinker. He was also a great friend, not just to me but to the entire community of autism families who adopted him as their own. Dan paid a heavy price in some circles for his conviction that the "age of autism" was an episode in history that had a clear beginning and a necessary end. But his many notable discoveries—from the Amish anomaly to the role of mercury poisoning in hysteria to the real identities of eight of the original Kanner eleven—will stand the test of time. He saved a lot of lives. We will miss him.

Mark Blaxill
Cambridge, MA
February 22, 2017